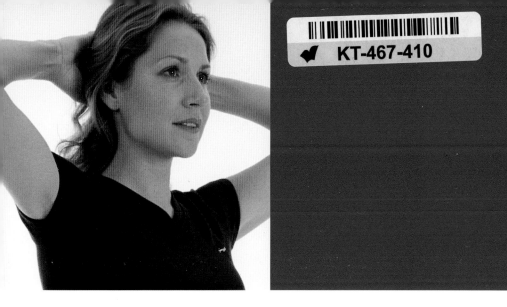

Back in Shape

the 10-week
post baby
recovery plan

Sally Lewis

hamlyn

1

Contents

Introduction

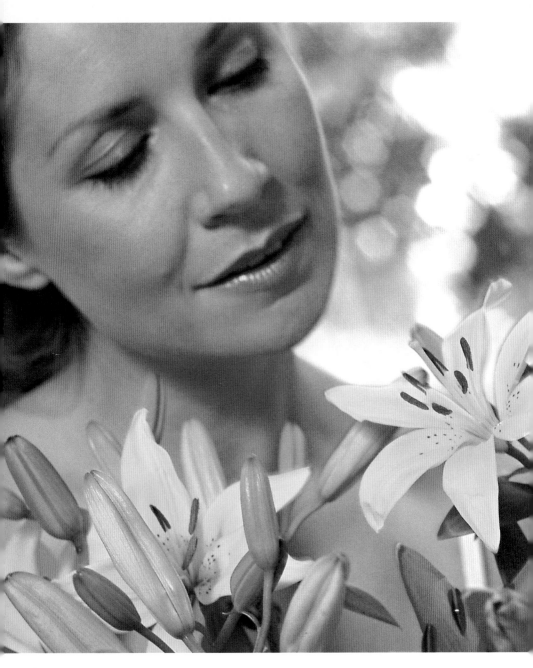

AFTER THE BIRTH

Having just had a baby, your body will have gone through many dramatic changes. The after-effects of these changes are looked at in detail to give you a greater insight into what has been happening to you physically, and to help dispel common anxieties and fears. Both conventional and complementary remedies are on offer to help alleviate pain and discomfort and to aid recovery in the early days after the birth.

DIET

A section on diet gives you practical advice on how to eat healthily in your new challenging circumstances, with recipes specifically developed to increase your energy levels without adding to your weight.

EXERCISE

Exercises are targeted at particular problem areas for postnatal mothers, and take into account the pain and physical weaknesses that are often a consequence of pregnancy and birth. Included are exercises that you can actually do with your baby to enable you to keep up your fitness training when you have no time to yourself.

WELLBEING

Beauty treatments and techniques are detailed, which aim to promote your general wellbeing – mental, spiritual and physical. These techniques will show you the value and importance of taking care of yourself during this vital stage in your life. There are therapies to cater for all your needs – to help you cope with all of the different demands that you now have to meet from day to day.

10-WEEK PLAN

A step-by-step 10-week plan sets out achievable goals for diet, exercise and relaxation, so that you can chart your progress and keep motivated. If events put you off course or set you back for a while, you can easily pick up the programme and carry on once more at a later date. And remember that the minute you begin to get back in shape, you are already on the path to success.

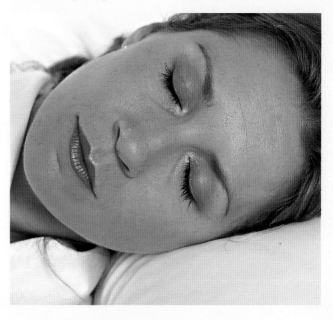

Remember that the minute you begin to **get back in shape,** you are already on the **path to success**!

After the birth

It is important to understand that after nine months of accommodating your growing baby, your body will have altered in shape. Expecting your body to return to normal a few days after the birth is unrealistic for most women; in fact, it can take up to a year for the body to be fully restored internally.

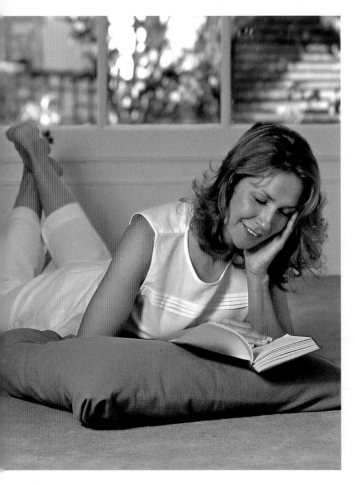

There will be changes in the way you feel and look after the birth of your baby. Mood swings, cravings, after-pains, sore breasts and headaches are the most common problems, along with the impact of stitches, fluid retention and stretch marks. This chapter gives advice on dealing with all of these.

The way you look

Perhaps the biggest shock for most women after birth is how their body looks. While you are likely to feel so much lighter and slimmer, you may be horrified at the loose skin that still hangs in folds. Crêpe-like skin is a common feature after birth, as is the excess bulge that lingers around the midriff. You may have lost your waist and feel that your thighs are heavier than before, and your breasts will also be considerably larger. With a little effort, however, you can make a big difference in your appearance, so be kind to yourself.

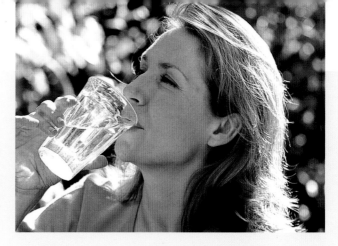

Drink plenty of water and herbal teas, particularly rosemary, as this improves the circulation

WEIGHT

In reality, having given birth you will have lost the weight of the baby, the placenta, the amniotic fluid and the membranes. During the next six weeks the uterus will shrink, and this will also cause you to lose weight. But the chances are that you will be heavier than you were before you became pregnant. Breast-feeding, eating the right types of food and taking exercise will all help with weight loss. This is not the time to worry about dieting.

STOMACH

The stomach will shrink after birth, but you will be left with some loose skin which only diet and exercise can combat. Specific spot exercises for the abdominal muscles will help tone and tighten the tummy (see pages 33, 34 and 42). Additionally a healthy diet will encourage the loss of fat from this area (see the chapter on Diet, pages 18–25).

BREASTS

Your breasts do not have any muscles and therefore ill-fitting garments or not wearing a bra will cause them to sag, particularly when you finish breast-feeding. The pectoral muscles that run under the breasts help support them and exercises can be carried out to strengthen these (see page 58). This is important because once the breasts are allowed to

drop they will not naturally come back into shape. Even if you decide not to breast-feed, it is still advisable to support your now larger breasts with a well-fitting bra. It is worth getting yourself measured at a reputable lingerie supplier, and once you have finished breast-feeding you will need another fitting, since your breasts will have changed from their pre-pregnancy days.

SKIN AND HAIR

Your skin and hair may have changed while you were pregnant – usually for the better – but many women experience problems after the birth. Skin generally becomes much drier, and you may find that you suffer some temporary hair loss. These occurrences can be deeply alarming but they are normal, so try not to worry. Instead, take positive steps to help your skin

and hair to recover. Spend time on caring for yourself wherever possible. In particular, treat your skin to a stimulating homemade facial or massage, which will also reinvigorate your whole system (see pages 78–79).

TO REPLENISH AND REVITALIZE SKIN AND HAIR

- Eat plenty of fruit and vegetables
- Drink herbal teas, particularly rosemary since this improves the circulation, and plenty of water
- Use a moisturizer on your face and all over your body
- Use a deep conditioner for your hair
- Make sure you get enough rest and sleep

The way you feel

Nothing can prepare you for having a baby, and for the emotions and confusion that you experience afterwards. One minute you will feel elated, the next miserable and depressed. Everything can become too much to cope with. Your body will feel as though it has been on the battlefield – it will even bear the scars! None of this is surprising considering you have only just emerged from an experience that is highly traumatic in every way.

You may want to discuss the birth with your partner or a close friend. Many women find that they need to relive it all, to try to understand the way it happened. Many memories will be a blur and you may want to put them in some sort of order. For some women, coming home from hospital can be terrifying and the thought of being alone daunting. Try to get someone to be around for a few days while you establish yourself back at home.

TIME-ALONE TIPS

- Try to rest whenever the baby sleeps.
- Lie down or use relaxation and meditation techniques at least once a day.
- Let the housework and other non-essential tasks go to give you some time to yourself.
- Do not be afraid to ask for help from members of your family or your partner, if they are not too busy.

'BABY BLUES'

Tears are very common, especially during the first week, and most mothers experience the 'baby blues' around the third to fifth day after the birth. You will probably find that the slightest thing sets you off, yet the tears go as quickly as they come. Do not let anyone tell you to pull yourself together. This is a very confusing and life-changing phase and it requires expression in whatever way is right for you. Sometimes just having the shoulder of a supportive partner, mother or friend is all that is required to make you feel better. Your partner may be more sympathetic and understanding if you can share your feelings with him, too. However, should you feel very depressed several weeks after birth, it is worth talking to your health visitor or doctor to rule out the possibility of postnatal depression. Bach Flower Remedies may help, as will herbal tonics. Unwinding during the stressful early days after the birth is essential: try relaxation, meditation or breathing techniques.

TIME FOR YOURSELF

Finding time for yourself is important and perhaps one of the most difficult things to achieve. You may find that you feel selfish and guilty yet desperately in need of some time alone or away from the baby. New arrivals generally mean all routines go out of the window, so expect to feel as if you are on call 24 hours a day. Being left alone for 30–40 minutes while you claim back some of yourself will bring huge benefits to everyone, not just to you.

> Nothing can prepare you for **having a baby,** and for the **emotions** and confusion that you experience afterwards

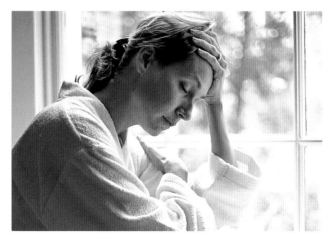

Postnatal problems

You may suffer from specific physical problems arising from delivery difficulties, as well as a range of nagging after-effects from both pregnancy and birth. These troublesome aches and sensations are a normal consequence of what your body has gone through and there are several simple measures you can take to make you feel better in the short term and speed up the healing process.

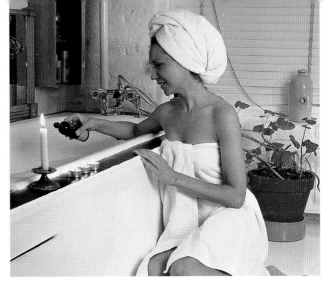

HEALING HELP

- **Arnica,** most effective for bruising, can be taken in homeopathic tablet form during labour; otherwise, take as soon as you can after the birth, continuing for at least a week.
- Apply **arnica, comfrey** or **calendula cream** externally.
- Soak in warm, salted baths or baths with a few drops of **lavender** or **chamomile essential** oils, or recommended blends of oils made up by a qualified aromatherapist.
- Apply **cold compresses** to reduce heat and swelling; use a packet of frozen peas or crushed ice wrapped in a soft towel.
- **Bach Flower Remedies** can help restore harmony to your emotions and, in turn, physical wellbeing.

Safety note: Never apply ice directly to the skin.

Soak in **warm salted baths** or baths to which a few drops of **lavender or chamomile** essential oils have been added

CAESAREAN BIRTHS

Caesarean births present their own pains and complications. You will feel sore and bruised, and very unenthusiastic about pulling yourself out of bed, but you must do so as soon as you can. Once up, your body will have the chance of helping to restore itself. Do not be surprised if you have excess bleeding. This is quite common, since the blood may well have pooled in the pelvic area during the Caesarean. The area around the scar can be massaged, but not over the stitches themselves until they have completely healed. Many stitches are dissolvable, but others may need to be removed by your midwife or doctor. Check which type you have before leaving hospital. After a shower, gently pat the area dry. Arnica homeopathic tablets will help to reduce the bruising, and aromatherapy and Bach Flower Remedies may also be effective.

A Caesarean birth will mean that your body takes longer to heal than with a natural delivery, and you should avoid any heavy lifting or strenuous work for six weeks. The upside is the pelvic floor will not have been damaged.

EPISIOTOMY

If you had an episiotomy or suffered a tear during the birth, you are bound to feel sore, especially around your stitches. The remedies effective for a Caesarean will also ease the pain and discomfort of an episiotomy or tear, as will warm, salted baths, and comfrey or calendula creams. Try to keep pressure off the area.

HAEMORRHOIDS

Another very common postnatal complaint is haemorrhoids, which occur when the blood vessels rupture during labour. For many women, constipation becomes a problem after birth, which can add to the likelihood of haemorrhoids developing through straining too hard during bowel movements. A diet that is high in fibre will help, as will massaging the abdomen with rosemary essential oil blended with a base oil, such as sweet almond oil (in the ratio of 1 drop essential oil to 1 teaspoon massage oil).

HEALING HELP

- Apply over-the-counter **haemorrhoid creams** or ointments; ask your health visitor or doctor to recommend the best kind to use.
- Apply cold compresses to the area; **chamomile** tea and **marigold** will reduce heat and help alleviate itching.
- Homeopathic remedies are effective – try **pulsatilla,** and **witch hazel** and **horsechestnut** cream.
- Add **frankincense, geranium** or **juniper** essential oils to your bathwater (follow instructions on the bottle for how much oil to use).
- **Reflexology** can aid in the treatment of both haemorrhoids and constipation.

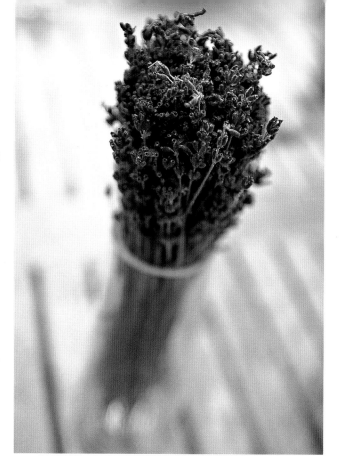

As for relieving after-pains, use **lavender essential oil** blended with **sweet almond oil**

AFTER-PAINS

After-pains are not generally felt after a first baby but may be experienced for some days after the birth of subsequent babies. They are caused by the shrinking of the uterus. While some women find them uncomfortable, others do not notice them. Bear in mind that these pains are occurring for a good purpose, so try to regard them in a positive light. If you find them particularly painful, take a dose of paracetamol or get your partner to give you a gentle massage with a base oil containing lavender essential oil.

BREAST DISCOMFORT

You can expect some discomfort from your breasts as the milk comes in, generally around the third day after the birth. As they swell with milk, you may find them heavy and uncomfortable. Additionally, you could experience a dragging sensation through them which is caused by the milk flow and the stimulation of your baby starting to feed. This is often known as the 'reflex' or 'let down'.

Breast-feeding stimulates contractions of the uterus, and these after-pains are caused by the production of the hormone oxytocin. Gentle abdominal massage may bring some relief, as well as relaxation during and after feeding. If you find the pain too great, a small dose of paracetamol may be worthwhile.

Drying up the milk supply
Should you decide to bottle-feed, your breast milk will take several days to dry up and you can experience some pain during that time as the milk is reabsorbed.

Mastitis Mastitis is a very painful inflammation of the breasts, with accompanying flu-like symptoms. Conventional treatment includes the use of antibiotics.

NATURAL REMEDY FOR **SORE BREASTS**

- Some women may find their breasts incredibly large, swollen, solid and sore when their milk first comes in. In this case, try placing the outside **leaves of a cabbage** inside your bra or warm flannels on the breasts. This will help draw out the heat and alleviate the pain. This is also an effective alternative treatment for mastitis.

SORE NIPPLES
Try to expose your nipples to the air after feeding. Do not scrub them in order to harden them. Make sure that the baby does not suck on the nipple itself but puts her jaws around the areola (the pigmented ring around the nipple) so that the nipple is drawn to the back of her mouth. Dry the nipples thoroughly after feeding and place breast pads inside your bra to soak up any excess milk that may be stimulated. Regularly feed your baby from both sides to enable the milk to drain through the ducts. Healing creams and homoeopathic remedies such as chamomilla, ignatia, pulsatilla, aconite, sulphur, graphites or silicea may help.

HEALING HELP

- Apply over-the-counter creams or ointments; ointment containing **calendula lotion** is particularly soothing and natural.
- Homeopathic treatments are effective, including **chamomilla**, **ignatia**, **pulsatilla**, **aconite**, **sulphur**, **graphites** and **silicea**.

ABDOMINAL DISCOMFORT
Massage is one of the best natural therapies available, and is particularly effective in aiding relaxation. It is very popular among some African tribes and is used for several weeks after birth, where other women will massage the postnatal mother. Massage

promotes mental and physical wellbeing in general, as well as specifically helping to shrink the uterus after the birth. As for relieving after-pains, use lavender essential oil blended with sweet almond oil for abdominal discomfort (see page 81)

FLUID RETENTION
This is another general discomfort. Although you will have lost a good deal of fluid at birth, you may still find yourself bloated and carrying excess weight. Drinking herbal tea, such as fennel, can have a cleansing effect, as can massage since this stimulates the lymph system and helps it to drain. You might also like to eat natural diuretics (see box, below).

NATURAL **DIURETICS**

- **Dandelion** – add the fresh leaves to a mixed leaf salad
- **Celery**
- **Parsley**
- **Fennel**
- **Asparagus**

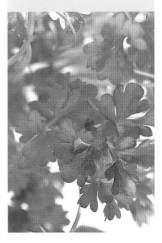

EXCESS SWEATING

From the moment of birth your body embarks on another set of changes as it grapples with an involuting uterus, milk production, a sore and bruised vagina or Caesarean scar and a return to the pre-pregnant state. Hormones change once again, too, and this may affect your mood and cause fluid retention. Excess sweating is common but take heart because it does help with reducing fluid and consequently weight loss.

TIREDNESS

Being overwhelmingly tired after the birth is almost universal. There is nothing that can adequately prepare you for the physical effort of labour and birth, and now you have the new demands of motherhood to contend with. But remember, these do not last a lifetime. With consideration and a little care, you should be able to catch up on sleep and take rests without feeling guilty. Using relaxation techniques and complementary treatments that promote general good health and exercising will all help. A herbal tonic obtained from a reputable herbalist can provide a necessary boost to restoring your wellbeing after the birth.

HEADACHES

Many women experience headaches for several weeks after birth. These are due to hormonal changes or strain during delivery. Some women experience headaches for 48 hours after an epidural. If you are breast-feeding your baby, you may wish to avoid conventional headache remedies.

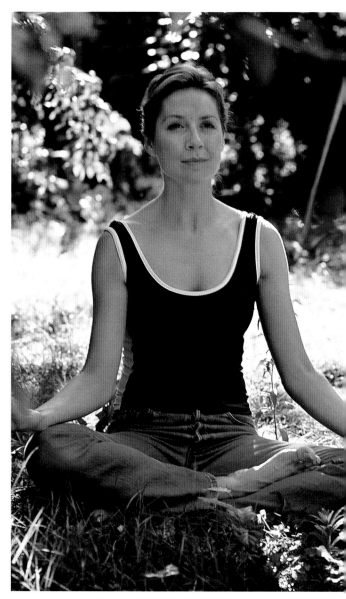

Breathing techniques can be **beneficial** since many headaches may be caused by **stress**

Massage relief Head and facial massage (see page 79) are extremely effective drug-free headache relief alternatives that release tension. You should be aware, in addition to your head, of any pent-up tension in your shoulders and neck area, and use massage to these areas to release it (see pages 78–79).

Aromatherapy Apply lavender or peppermint oil to the temples. When massaging oil into the temples (see page 78), blend with a massage oil (in the ratio of 1 drop essential oil to 1 teaspoon massage oil). Try inhalations of lavender, peppermint or eucalyptus oil either by using an essential oil burner or by putting a few drops of the oil on a handkerchief and holding it over your face and breathing in.

Other alternative treatments Breathing techniques can be beneficial (see page 32), since many headaches may be caused by stress. Relaxation and meditation techniques will also help. Reflexology is another recommended therapy for headaches, in which pressure points on the big toe are targeted.

Rehydration Headaches are often a symptom of dehydration: you may not realize how much fluid loss you need to compensate for following the birth. You also need to increase your fluid intake if you are breast-feeding. Drink filtered or bottled mineral water – at room temperature as opposed to being ice cold. Limit your intake of tea and coffee, since too much caffeine can have a dehydrating effect. Drink herbal teas instead, particularly fennel, strong chamomile and rosemary.

STRETCH MARKS

Stretch marks that have occurred during pregnancy will shrink and become less obvious with time. Ideally, you will have been massaging them with oil while pregnant. Again, a massage oil containing lavender oil is an effective treatment for stretch marks. Mandarin and tangerine oils are also worth trying. Remember to read the instructions on the bottles regarding quantities and how to use the oils, or consult an aromatherapist.

Head and facial massage are **effective** drug-free alternatives that **release tension**

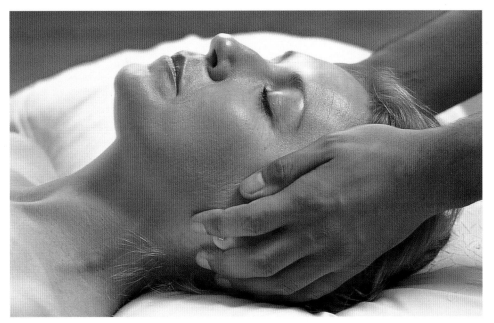

FOOD CRAVINGS

Food cravings can develop after birth, especially if you are breast-feeding. You may find that you become suddenly overwhelmingly hungry. The physical demands being made on you will quickly deplete your energy levels. Your blood sugar levels may be slightly erratic in the first few weeks after birth as your body struggles to reassert itself into a new routine. All this means that you will find yourself reaching out for the nearest available snack. Stock up with readily available healthy snacks to stop yourself eating biscuits, crisps and sweets. Work out when during the day you feel most hungry and try to rearrange your day so you can move your main meal to this time.

HEALTHY **SNACKS**

- Slices of **wholemeal bread**
- **Porridge oats**
- **Rice cakes**
- **Fresh fruit**, particularly bananas, which slowly release sugar into the bloodstream
- **Raw vegetables**
- **Nuts**

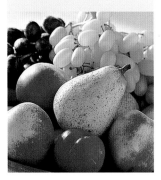

HERBAL TONICS

A herbal tonic is an effective remedy for lethargy, tiredness, minor depression, tearfulness and stress. There are several herbal tonics now available to purchase directly over the counter – a reputable health shop or pharmacy that specializes in alternative products will advise you. Alternatively, consult a herbalist.

> One of the easiest ways to **ingest herbs** is to make herbal teas

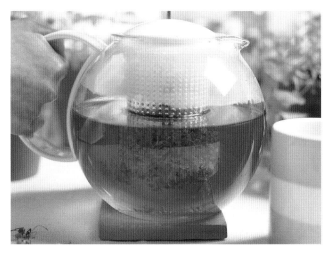

HERBAL TEAS

One of the easiest ways to ingest herbs is to make herbal teas. If you are breast-feeding, you can pass on the benefits of the following herbs through your breast milk to your baby.

- **Chamomile** is a relaxant and so a good bedtime drink.
- **Peppermint** can aid digestion. If your baby is experiencing wind or colic, drink a cup of peppermint tea before the next feed.
- **Celery seed** aids milk flow for breast-feeding mothers.

- **Lemonbalm tea** with a teaspoon of honey added can help new mothers regain their strength after birth.
- **Raspberry leaf** tea, which is thought to strengthen the womb in the last three months of pregnancy, can also help to restore womb tone after the birth.
- The **common nettle** is wonderful for its tonic qualities, particularly for nursing mothers, since it promotes iron levels and aids a good milk supply. Drink in tea form or eat raw.

THERAPIES FOR **POSTNATAL PROBLEMS**

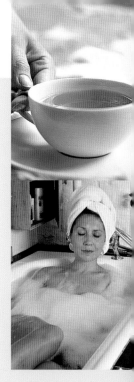

PROBLEMS	REMEDIES
Excess weight	Healthy diet and exercise
Skin and hair	Diet; herbal teas – rosemary; water; herbal treatments; facials and beauty treatments; massage
'Baby blues'	Bach Flower Remedies; herbal tonics; relaxation, meditation and breathing techniques
Caesarean births	Arnica homeopathic tablets; herbal baths; aromatherapy; Bach Flower Remedies
Episiotomy	Arnica homeopathic tablets; comfrey and calendula creams; warm, salted baths; aromatherapy – lavender and chamomile essential oils; cold compresses
After-pains	Massage with lavender essential oil, blended with a base oil
Breast discomfort	Cabbage leaves to extract heat; abdominal massage
Sore nipples	Healing creams; homeopathic – chamomilla, ignatia, pulsatilla, aconite, sulphur, graphites, silicea
Abdominal discomfort	Massage with lavender essential oil, blended with a base oil
Fluid retention	Herbal teas – fennel; diet – dandelion leaves, celery, parsley, fennel, asparagus
Headaches	Head massage – lavender or peppermint essential oils applied to the temples; facial exercises; inhalations; breathing, relaxation and meditation techniques; reflexology; filtered or mineral water; herbal teas
Stretch marks	Massage with lavender, mandarin or tangerine essential oils, blended with a base oil
Food cravings	Diet – wholesome foods and healthy snacks such as fruit and raw vegetables; more frequent, smaller meals; move main meal time to when most hungry

Diet

Now that your baby has arrived, it is important to consider your food needs. Food has a direct effect on the condition of the body and your general feeling of wellbeing. To keep healthy and enable the body to fight disease and infection, as well as to cope with the increased demands of having a baby, you have to feed it the right types of food.

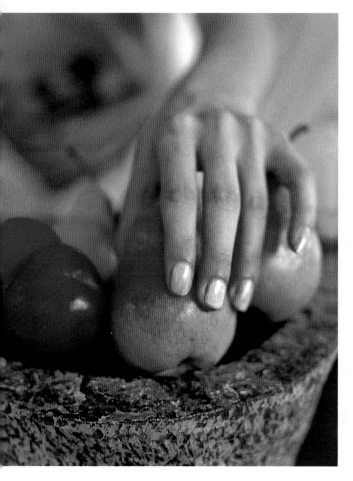

MAINTAINING THE HEALTHY HABIT

It is often said that you are what you eat, and during pregnancy you probably took great care over your diet. That same attitude should be maintained after the birth. A diet that is properly balanced is the only way to ensure that your body receives the appropriate amount and range of nutrients to achieve optimum health.

NUTRITIONAL NEEDS

After the birth, your body will once again be going through a period of dramatic change – mental and physical, including hormonal. Diet can play an important role in assisting it to deal with these changes. Finding time for shopping and preparing fresh foods becomes more difficult and the simplest, easiest option is to eat processed pre-packed meals from the freezer. Yet this is likely to have a direct adverse effect on your health.

So what are nutritional needs? They are the types of food that we need to eat to maintain, restore and build our immune system. They give us energy, create new cells and provide us with a healthy body. We all need proteins, fats and carbohydrates, as well as vitamins and minerals. We also need water, which is found in most foods and makes up a large proportion of our body. Good sources of fibre should be included because it is vital for a healthy digestive system.

Healthy choices

Your diet should include some fresh fruit, vegetables or salads every day. Meat and fish that is fresh should ideally be used instead of frozen or pre-packed. The processes that are used to preserve fresh food can mean that certain nutrients are lost. However, frozen vegetables are the exception to the rule, since they retain their vitamins and minerals. Choose organic foods where possible.

Refined foods have some of their nutrients removed during the refining process. This process also destroys the food's natural fibre content, making the product less easily digested. Sugar, white rice and white bread are all refined food products and as such are best avoided.

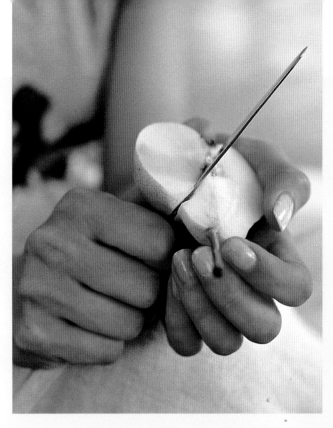

Food has a **direct effect** on the condition of the body and the general feeling of **wellbeing**

Include in your diet one serving a day of milk, cheese or another dairy product; two servings of protein – meat, fish, poultry, nuts, beans, peas or lentils; four servings of complex carbohydrates, such as wholemeal bread, brown rice, pasta, potatoes or muesli and five servings of fruit, vegetables or salads. If you are breast-feeding, increase your intake of dairy produce by at least another portion and add a little extra fat.

A balanced diet

The modern world has created environmental and psychological stresses that take their toll on our bodies, potentially lowering our resources. With the widespread use of pesticides, intensive farming methods, hormones, preservatives and additives in the growing and preparation of our food, our diets can be deficient in the nutrients required to cope with these increased demands.

Foods for life

To ensure that your diet offers the correct nutritional content, you need to know a little about which foods fit into the different food groups that form the basis of a balanced diet, what function they fulfil and what proportion of your overall diet each food group needs to make up.

PROTEINS

Nutritional requirement: 15 per cent of your daily diet.
Proteins are the body's building blocks. All the main organs of the body are created from protein. Skin, hair and bone can also contain protein. When large amounts of protein are eaten, the body stores the excess in muscles and organs. Insufficient protein causes the body's metabolism to slow down. Found in meat, fish and poultry, protein can also be provided in the diet by eating nuts and pulses (beans, peas and lentils).

CARBOHYDRATES

Nutritional requirement: 60 per cent of your daily diet.
Carbohydrates are the body's main source of energy and they come in several forms. The simplest, known as simple carbohydrates, are fructose and glucose, otherwise commonly known as sugar. Complex carbohydrates are found in vegetables, cereals and some fruits. They take longer to be broken down than the simple sugars do and are consequently more beneficial since they release energy at a slower rate.

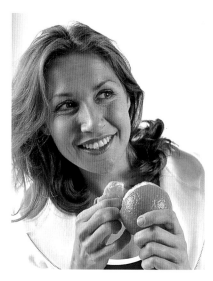

Your diet should include **fresh fruit, vegetables** and **salads** every day

HEALTHY ALTERNATIVES

- Use **low-fat spread** or **polyunsaturated margarine** instead of butter.
- Choose **low-fat alternatives** for full-fat dairy products, such as cream, full-fat milk and cheeses, for example **semi-skimmed** or **skimmed milk, low-fat yogurt** or **low-fat fromage frais.**
- Eat **lean meat, chicken** and **turkey** rather than fatty meat products, such as pies and sausages. Also, try **reduced-fat sausages.**
- Eat more **fish**, especially **oily fish.**
- Use **monounsaturated** or **polyunsaturated oils**, such as **olive, corn** or **soya oil** instead of lard or butter.
- Create homemade salad dressings. Replace mayonnaise or salad cream with **olive oil** and add herbs for flavourings.
- For special occasions or treats make **low-fat biscuits** or **cakes,** but do not treat as everyday food. Replace high-fat snacks, such as crisps, chocolate, cakes, pastries and biscuits, with **fresh** or **dried fruit, breadsticks** and **vegetables** cut into sticks.
- Fill up on starchy food, such as **pasta, rice** and **potatoes. Baked potatoes** or **boiled** are best. **Couscous** is another healthy carbohydrate alternative.
- **Grill, steam, bake** or **microwave** food whenever possible instead of frying. Roast meat on a rack so that the fat drips away.
- Use **heavy-based** or **nonstick pans.** This way, you do not have to add fat when cooking to prevent food from sticking.

FATS

Nutritional requirement: 25–30 per cent of your daily diet. Another source of energy, fats provide twice as many calories as proteins or carbohydrates for the same amount of weight. As such, these are usually the culprits in excess weight gain. Particularly fattening are saturated fats – butter, cheese and cream. However, other fats are nutritionally beneficial, for example polyunsaturated fats, which can be found in nuts, oils and seeds.

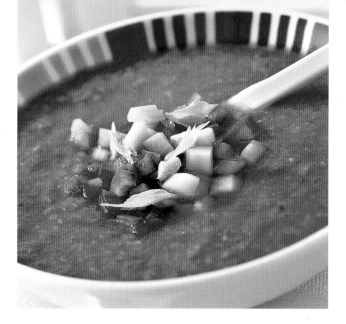

Homemade soups will be **nutritious** as well as filling

ANTIOXIDANTS

- The main antioxidants are **vitamins C** and **E,** and **betacarotene,** which the body turns into **vitamin A.** Known as **'ACE' vitamins,** they are believed to promote good health and protect against disease by aiding the body's natural defences against damage by free radicals.
- Antioxidants are provided in the diet by **dark green** leafy vegetables (such as **broccoli** and **spinach**); **yellow-orange fruits** and **vegetables** (such as **carrots, apricots, mangoes, sweet potatoes** and **red peppers**); **citrus fruits; wholemeal bread** and **pasta; avocados** and **vegetable oils.**

VITAMINS AND MINERALS

These are essential in maintaining the body's metabolic function and are found in most foods (see the chart summarizing the Essential Vitamins and Minerals on pages 22–23). Eating a varied, balanced diet will help eliminate the need to take vitamin and mineral supplements.

FIBRE

Fibre is necessary for the disposal of waste from the body. Fibrous foods include wholemeal bread; rice; cereals (e.g. bran flakes and muesli); wholemeal pasta; vegetables (e.g. cabbage, peas and potatoes); fresh fruit (e.g. bananas and raspberries); dried fruit (e.g. dried apricots and stewed prunes); nuts and pulses (e.g. butter beans).

FOODS TO **AVOID**

- Foods high in **saturated fats, sugar, cholesterol, refined sugars** and **animal products,** including **biscuits, cakes** and **pastries,** which cause blood sugar to rise and dip quickly, thereby inducing tiredness.
- **Alcohol** also affects blood sugar and depletes vitamins B and C. It is also highly dehydrating and can damage the skin.
- High levels of **cholesterol** are found in **hard cheese** and **full-fat dairy products.**
- Highly processed '**junk' foods** and **fizzy drinks** are low in nutrients and high in additives.

143951 diet **21**

Soothing foods

Eating foods rich in carbohydrates will ensure that your brain produces serotonin, a calming substance. These foods include potatoes, parsnips, turnips, pasta, bread, lentils and kidney beans as well as rice and pulses. Bony fish (e.g. sardines), yogurt, milk, cheese, dried apricots, dark green leafy vegetables, nuts and seeds all provide serotonin and calcium.

Energy-giving foods

Most foodstuffs provide you with energy, but certain types of food give you more energy than others. When broken down in the body, these foods slowly release sugar into the bloodstream, thus ensuring that the blood sugars are stabilized. High-energy foods include wholemeal bread, cereal or cereal bars, rice cakes, porridge oats and oat biscuits, brown rice, pasta, potatoes, fruit (e.g. apples, bananas and pears) and dried fruit (e.g. apricots, dates and figs).

HIGH-ENERGY DRINKS
Freshly squeezed fruit and vegetable juices make quick and easy energy drinks. They contain a range of vitamins and minerals, including the all-important antioxidants, and are easily broken down and absorbed into

ESSENTIAL **VITAMINS AND MINERALS**

NUTRIENTS	FOOD SOURCES	BENEFITS
Vitamin A	Liver; eggs; carrots; spinach; broccoli; fruit	Eyesight; skin; possible protection against cancer; antioxidant
Vitamin C	Peppers; oranges; strawberries; blackcurrants	Helps heal wounds; may fight infections; protects gums; keeps joints and ligaments in good working order; antioxidant
Vitamin D	Green leafy vegetables; corn; avocado; asparagus; wheatgerm; wholegrain cereals; brown rice; pure vegetable oils; nuts; seeds; soya beans; tofu	Cell growth; antioxidant
Vitamin B1	Most foods including wheatgerm; wholegrain cereals; pulses; nuts	Helps the breakdown of carbohydrates; nervous system
Vitamin B2	Liver; kidney; dairy produce;eggs; brewer's yeast; wheat bran; wheatgerm	Repairs body tissue
Vitamin B3	Fish; wheatgerm; wholegrain cereals	Essential for chemical reactions
Vitamin B6	Lean meat; liver; fish; wholegrains; bananas; avocados; potatoes	Nervous system; skin; red blood cells
Vitamin B12	Liver; kidney; some fish; shellfish; eggs; milk	Blood and nerves

Fresh fruit and vegetable juices are **delicious** and offer real **health benefits**

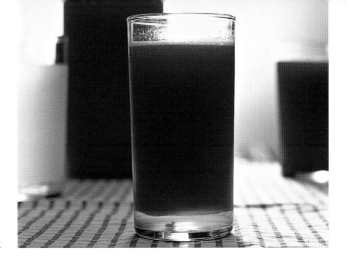

the system. Among their health benefits are improved energy levels, boosted immune system and restored vitality. Fresh juices are both cleansing and nourishing.

ESSENTIAL **VITAMINS AND MINERALS**

NUTRIENTS	FOOD SOURCES	BENEFITS
Vitamin K	Most vegetables, especially dark green leafy ones; liver	Helps in the production of some proteins
Calcium	Red meat; liver; oily fish; wholegrain cereals; leafy green vegetables **NB**: Breast-feeding mothers need extra calcium	Bones, teeth and nails; muscles and nerve function
Zinc	Red meat; sardines; shellfish; root vegetables; nuts; seeds	Boosts immune system; improves red blood cells
Iron	Lean red meat; liver; pulses; dark green leafy vegetables; dried fruit	Makes haemoglobin, the pigment in red blood cells that helps transport oxygen around the body
Selenium	Lean meat; liver; fish; shellfish; brazil nuts; wholegrain cereals; tomatoes broccoli; onions	Regulates thyroid hormones and protects against artery clogging; cancels out the pollutants in the body
Magnesium	Lean meat; fish; shellfish; pulses; brown rice; green vegetables; bananas; nuts; seeds	Keeps up energy levels – releases energy from the muscles; stops blood sugar fluctuations which can cause dizziness and tiredness; needed for production of cells, bone, proteins and fatty acids
Potassium	Bananas; citrus fruits; dried fruits; nuts; seeds; potatoes; pulses	Maintains normal blood pressure and regular heartbeat; facilitates transmission of nerve impulses

Avoiding weight gain

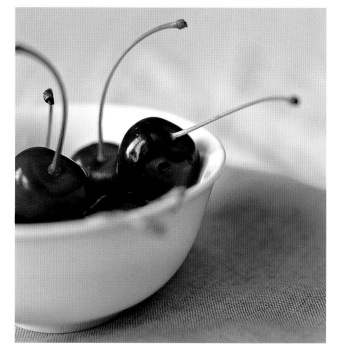

After the birth of your baby, you will probably weigh more than you did before pregnancy. Do not despair – a sensible eating plan combined with a steady exercise programme will help you achieve the results you desire. But be realistic. You spent nine months carrying and growing a baby, so do not expect excess weight to disappear overnight.

Do not start snacking on convenience foods for an instant energy boost, as these generally provide little nutritional value while being high in calories. Raising the blood-sugar levels quickly will also cause them to plummet subsequently, and you will then need another quick fix to sustain that energetic feeling.

LOSE WEIGHT GRADUALLY
Aim to lose about 0.5 kg/1 lb a week. That may sound a small amount, but this way you will be able to keep to your healthy diet and maintain your weight loss. Gradual weight loss is the

Snack on **fruit** rather than the **'empty calories'** of convenience foods

healthier way to restore your body shape.

Eat regularly – missing meals is not a healthy way to lose weight. If breast-feeding, you may experience constant hunger pangs. Small regular meals will help to keep these at bay. Do not worry if, for a few months, you find yourself needing five small meals a day. Providing they are healthy, you will still lose weight.

Energy foods, that is the complex carbohydrates, will also be important. Select foods listed under Energy-giving Foods on page 22 and Foods for Life on pages 20–21 to make up a diet that boosts your energy levels several times throughout the day.

Do not try crash diets or new diet fads. They may depress you in the long term and prevent you from getting vital nutrients.

TIPS FOR **HEALTHY WEIGHT LOSS**

- Increase **fibre-rich** foods such as **fruit, vegetables, wholegrains, beans** and **lentils. Fruit** and **vegetables** are also **high in vitamins** but low in fats.
- Choose **low-fat dairy products** but keep up your dairy intake, especially if you are breast-feeding.
- Eat **fish, poultry** and **lean meat.** Avoid frying food. Cut down on fatty meat products such as sausages, sausage rolls and pork pies.
- Reserve pastries, cakes and biscuits for special occasions.
- **Enjoy your food!** There is a lot to be gained from it.

WEIGHT-CONTROL DIET

BREAKFAST
Choose from:

Porridge oats or fortified **breakfast cereal** with semi-skimmed milk and a **serving of fruit**. Consider adding sliced banana to your cereal; the slow release of sugar will be very beneficial.

A bowl of fruit including dried fruit and natural yogurt.

Wholemeal toast with a scraping of polyunsaturated margarine and low-sugar jam or marmalade.

Serve **tea, herbal tea, water** or **fruit juice** with any of the above. Try hot water with a slice of lemon for a refreshing and cleansing drink.

MID-MORNING
Choose from:

A **banana**, a **bowl of fruit**, a **cereal snack bar**, a **handful of nuts** and **raisins** or a few **rice cakes**.

LUNCH
Choose from:

A **bowl of home-made soup** with a slice of wholemeal bread (no spread).

A **bowl of pasta** with vegetables, chicken or fish in a tomato or vegetable sauce. Do not use cream, full-fat milk or butter in the sauce.

A **wholemeal sandwich** made from two slices of wholemeal bread filled with salad and tuna, chicken, cottage cheese or low-fat cheese spread. Use a scraping of polyunsaturated margarine but do not add mayonnaise or salad cream.

A **bowl of salad** including raw vegetables, such as raw carrot, onion or celery. You can add a proprietary low-calorie dressing or make your own. Use vegetables that are in season, adding variety and colour.

AFTERNOON TREAT
Choose from:

Fresh fruit; dried fruit; a **cereal snack bar**; a **plain biscuit**; **rice cakes** with a scraping of **peanut butter**.

DINNER
Choose from:

Pasta or **baked potato** with chicken or fish and vegetables.

Rice with chicken, fish, seafood or egg.

Fruit dessert, which could be stewed, baked or grilled if wished. Drizzle a small amount of sugar and yogurt over it and you will not feel you are missing out.

Exercise

There is no avoiding the fact that after the birth of your baby, you will need to invest time and energy to get your body back in shape. The changes that your body has gone through will not be reversed overnight, but with the right attention your body shape will improve.

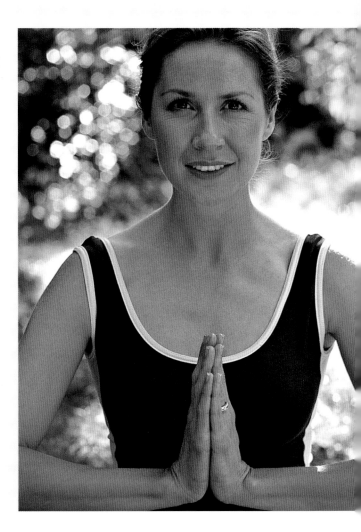

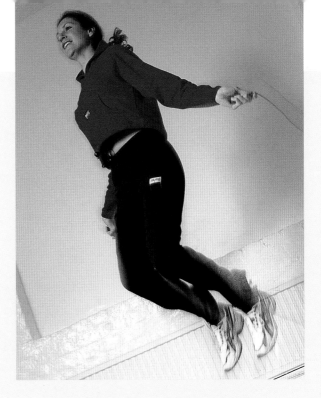

Exercising gives you more energy, and gradually it will become part of your everyday routine and way of life

At first, you are likely to feel that you cannot find the time or the enthusiasm to exercise. But the sooner you begin, the easier it will become. Exercise gives you more energy, and gradually it will become part of your everyday routine and way of life. At a time when many demands are being placed on you, exercise will keep you motivated and create a general feeling of wellbeing.

HOW THE EXERCISES WORK

The simple exercises presented here are designed to work the areas of your body affected by pregnancy and are achievable whether you have never exercised before or were a committed workout enthusiast prior to becoming pregnant. You can always increase the intensity of the exercise programme, but start off slowly and take your time, building up your strength and stamina as you go.

The idea is to work all of the body to gain the maximum amount of benefit. Do not be tempted to think that your upper body does not need as much attention as your abdominals do. Having toned, strong arms and strong back muscles will define your shape.

TIGHTENING YOUR STOMACH

Obviously you will feel that your abdominal muscles, more than any others, need attention. The exercises which follow that work specifically on your stomach will indeed help you to gain control of and tighten those muscles that have been stretched. Some women find that their stomach muscles actually become tighter than they used to be in their pre-pregnant days.

STRENGTHENING YOUR BACK

Another consideration is your back. It will have suffered during pregnancy and must be strengthened. No stomach exercise will have the desired effect if your back is slouched and shoulders rounded. Many back problems stem from poor posture, and this commonly occurs during pregnancy with the increased weight from the growing foetus. Furthermore, carrying around a new baby and her equipment will continue to put strain on your back. Exercises to improve posture as well as tone and build the muscles of the back will help to avoid damage and prevent backache. Complementary therapists who use exercises such as the Alexander Technique and Pilates (see page 30) recognize the importance of posture and a straight back for overall good health and strength.

IMPROVING YOUR CARDIOVASCULAR SYSTEM

Toning exercises are only one of the types of exercise you need in order to bring about changes to your body. Aerobic work enhances your cardiovascular system and raises your metabolic rate. Increasing your heart rate is achieved through exercise that makes you breathe more heavily or pant. In this way you will burn up the fat stores that may be left over from pregnancy. Aerobic exercise will then help to keep any weight gain at bay. When you begin, you may find that your aerobic levels are low, but do not be discouraged. They will soon

> Some women find that their **stomach muscles** actually become **tighter** than in their pre-pregnant days

become higher as you exercise and you will be able to notice the difference. The increase in oxygen supply to the muscles will enable them to work more efficiently and the increase in your heart rate will aid stamina.

MAXIMIZING THE BENEFITS

Exercise should be fun. If it is not, it will become just another chore and you will be more likely to try and find excuses not to do it. The programme here is based on exercising every day, but you do not have to stick to this rigidly. You will need to exercise at least three times a week or you will fail to see any benefits. Try all the different types of exercise, since this gives you scope to choose the ones you like best. You can then adapt them to suit your programme. To achieve the all-over effect, however, you need to combine toning and aerobic work with stretching. There is a wide range of aerobic activities to choose from. Walking, skipping, jogging and dancing, along with sports such as netball, squash, hockey, basketball, swimming and cycling, are all forms of aerobic exercise, but gentle swimming will not have the desired effect – you need to raise your heart rate and breathe heavily.

> Exercises to **improve posture** as well as **tone and build** the muscles of the back will help to **avoid damage** and prevent backache

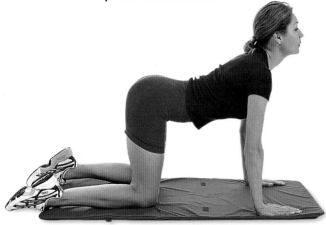

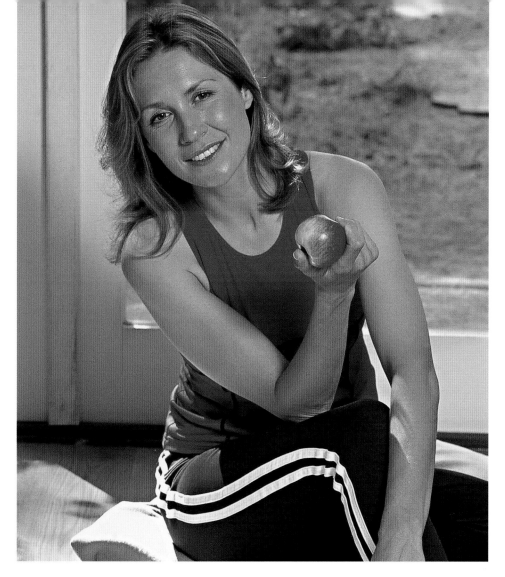

PROTECTION AND SAFETY

- **Wear appropriate clothing** when exercising. Anything easy and comfortable such as leggings and a T-shirt will be suitable, but remember to support your bust with a well-fitting bra or sports bra. This is particularly important after the birth of a baby. A towel or exercise mat will help to protect your knees and hip joints. You will also need a good pair of trainers for aerobic work.

- **To exercise safely**, you need to make sure that you do not rush the exercises or movements.

Warming up before your exercise routine and stretching before and after (see pages 38–43) will ensure that the muscles do not ache by helping to disperse any build-up of lactic acid that may collect in the muscles.

TYPES OF **EXERCISE**

AEROBICS
This type of exercise increases the heart rate and the supply of oxygen to the muscles. It will make you breathe harder.

Aerobic activities:
jogging, skipping, running, cycling, walking, rebounder, step and most sports.

KEY BENEFITS:
- increases the heart rate
- increases the supply of oxygen to the muscles
- boosts the metabolism
- builds stamina
- helps reduce weight by burning fat over a sustained period
- uses up extra calories

PILATES
This currently popular system of body maintenance coordinates body, mind and spirit. It works on the theory of naturally correct postural alignment.

KEY BENEFITS:
- lengthens short muscles and strengthens weak ones
- improves the quality of movement
- focuses on the core postural muscles to stabilize the body
- works to place the breath correctly
- aids mental relaxation

ALEXANDER TECHNIQUE
This is a therapy based upon the posture of the body, in particular the back. It teaches you how to realign your body and make changes to your daily positions, such as sitting, standing and bending down, to maintain good posture.

KEY BENEFITS:
- corrects posture
- improves quality of movement
- lengthens muscles
- improves energy flow
- aids mental relaxation

T'AI CHI
A series of slow-moving, concentrated movements carried out in conjunction with controlled breathing. These exercises coordinate body, mind and soul. They relax and de-stress, and enable you to retune into your inner energy.

KEY BENEFITS:
- uncovers your natural energy
- promotes mind and body control
- builds stamina and strength
- aids mental relaxation

YOGA
Yoga works on developing muscles and building strength and stamina through stretches. The use of correct breathing throughout these stretches harmonizes the mind and body. It can be a very tough form of exercise that places great demands on the muscles.

KEY BENEFITS:
- increases mobility in the joints and muscles
- develops the coordination of muscles
- increases mind–body awareness
- increases stamina
- increases strength
- aids relaxation

Your posture

Perhaps the biggest change you need to make before you begin any exercise is to check your posture. Poor posture will have very negative results – it will adversely affect the way in which you carry your body and how you use it. Standing straight improves your breathing, allowing plenty of oxygen to be sent to the muscles so that they work effectively.

POSTURE EXERCISE PROGRAMMES

Pilates, Alexander Technique and yoga (see opposite) focus on posture and the positive effects of breathing. Correct posture improves the balance between the mind and the body, giving it strength and stamina. Stretching exercises will enable you to become aware of your back and the way in which you carry it, but begin with the simple body check given on the right.

Circulation to the breasts

While the breasts themselves do not contain any muscle tissue, they do have muscles above and below which support them. Opening the chest, pushing back the shoulders and standing straight will help lift the chest and therefore hold the breasts up. Toning the pectoral muscles that support the breast tissue will also help support the breasts (see page 58). Exercises such as press-ups will also help here (see page 46), or simple exercises with weights (see page 49). Once the

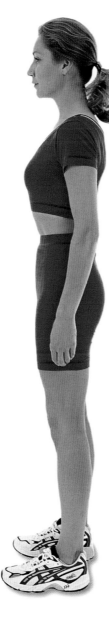

1 Stand in front of a long mirror, sideways on, with your feet hip-width apart.
2 Make sure that both your legs are facing front.
3 Do not lock the knees but keep the legs straight.
4 Allow the arms to rest naturally at your sides.
5 Check that your back is straight with shoulders dropped back and down and your hips not pushed forwards. You should be able to feel the pull of gravity on your spine. There should be no tension in your shoulders or back.
6 Feel your weight being supported by the middle of each foot. Do not rock back on to your heels or place your weight on the balls of your feet.

chest is open, the circulation improves. Learning to breathe deeply will also improve the circulation to the breast area (see Breathing Technique panel, page 32). Massaging around the breasts is also very useful, and particularly so if you are breast-feeding.

Breast-feeding techniques

Be aware of your posture during breast-feeding. Sitting with the back unsupported and allowing the shoulders to roll forwards will cause you to slouch, restricting the blood supply. The baby needs to be supported on a pillow or cushion and your back should also be supported and straight. Make sure that your feet are not reaching for the floor. If you find that your legs are a little short,

place them flat on a small stool or telephone directory, keeping your feet hip-width apart. Feed from both breasts to stimulate the milk flow. If you are uncomfortable with breast-feeding at first, you can lie down with the baby beside you. This takes the strain out of the back. Once you are confident with the process, try breathing in the way described in the panel while sitting or lying down. It is important to remember to keep the shoulders and the jaw relaxed throughout.

BREATHING TECHNIQUE

Practise this technique at different times throughout the day. You will find it particularly useful if you feel yourself becoming uptight or stressed. Breathing in this way for several minutes has a calming influence. Once you have mastered the art, you will be able to use it at any time. To begin with, practise the breathing technique while standing.

1 With feet hip-width apart and arms loose by your sides, check your posture. Your back should be straight, shoulders relaxed but feeling stretched downwards and chest open.
2 **Inhale** through your nose and feel the air travel down to your lungs. Allow them to open and expand sideways. Feel the tension in the lungs as you increase the amount of oxygen to them.

3 **Hold the breath** for a count of five.
4 **Release** the breath, and as you **exhale**, let the jaw drop forward and down. Allow the jaw to stretch and push the air out of the lungs until you feel that there is absolutely no more left. You will be amazed how much air is **exhaled**. The mouth should be open and relaxed and you will hear the breath as you e**xhale**.
5 **Relax** for a moment before you repeat the whole process again.
6 Try this **breathing** for **five breaths** and then rest. You should feel relaxed and restored.

Caesarean births

Caesarean births can cause different problems. While the pelvic floor muscles will not have been stretched and strained, your abdominal muscles have been cut through and are bruised and sore. It is important for you to become motivated and get moving as quickly as possible after the birth, even though you may initially find this a little frightening. Many women when they get up after having a Caesarean, bleed quite heavily from the vagina. This is quite usual, since the blood from the placenta and uterus can collect in this area. Talk over any anxieties you may have with your midwife, health visitor or doctor, who will be able to reassure you. As soon as you can get up on to your feet and start walking, do so. The body will benefit from the activity and you need to get the circulation going again as quickly as possible. Remember, though, not to lift anything heavy for six weeks. Once you feel more active, you can begin your exercise programme. The sooner you start, the better.

> After a Caesarean birth you will not be able to do any **heavy lifting** for six weeks

EXERCISES FOR **CAESAREAN BIRTHS**

The **first exercises** that you should start with are the **ankle rotations** (see page 37). You can do these easily while lying on the bed.

Follow with the **pelvic tilting** (see page 36) and **pelvic floor exercises** (see page 34), even though your pelvic floor has not been stretched as it would have

been in a normal delivery. You should also check the **rectus muscle** to see whether any distension has occurred (see page 35).

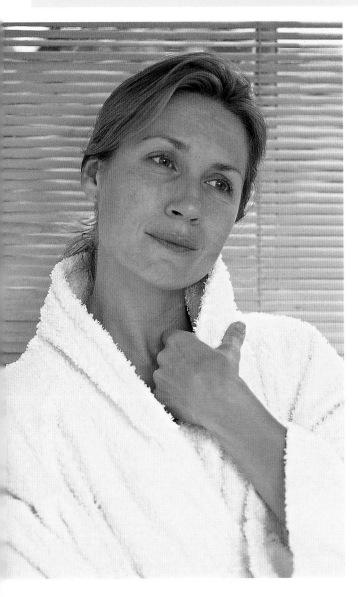

WHEN TO START ABDOMINAL EXERCISES

You will certainly need to wait until your wound has healed before you begin abdominal exercises, but you can perform abdominal retractions (see page 36) once the initial pain has gone from the site of the incision. At first, the thought of getting up from bed, coughing or sneezing may make you feel nervous. Place your hands over your wound to support it as you perform these functions and try to relax. If you have any specific worries, wait until your six-week postnatal check-up and consult your health adviser or doctor.

Once you have had your postnatal check-up, you should be ready to begin the other abdominal exercises. It may take longer with some of these exercises before you can increase the number of repetitions. Work at your own pace and ensure that you follow the exercises slowly and thoughtfully, really concentrating on your stomach muscles and your breathing as you do them. You will probably be about two weeks behind in your recovery compared to someone who has had a normal delivery, which means that the exercise programme will commence two weeks later for you.

Pelvic floor exercises

Hopefully, you will have been doing these throughout pregnancy. The pelvic floor muscles will be stretched if you have had a normal delivery and initially will be sore, but these exercises should be started as soon as possible. Encouraging the blood supply to the area will help cell regrowth and repair. The pelvic floor muscles will tighten and prevent any leaks that may result from coughing, sneezing or sudden bursts of activity.
Pelvic floor exercises should be performed daily, ideally several times a day. They are easy to do and you can do them anywhere you please, from standing at the sink to lying in bed.

FLUID **INTAKE**

- You must **drink more water** when you exercise. Get into the habit of reaching for the water bottle before anything else. Water keeps the body hydrated and cleans the system, flushing out the toxins that can make it sluggish.

FINDING YOUR **PELVIC FLOOR MUSCLE**

Try this simple exercise when urinating. Pull up and squeeze the internal muscles to stop the flow of urine mid-stream. If you find that it is not possible to control the flow at this stage, try the exercise at the beginning of urination or at the end. Gradually work towards stopping the flow midway. You should not need to squeeze any other muscles. Once you have mastered this, the exercises can be performed anywhere. No one will be able to tell that you are doing them. They can also be used during sexual intercourse, which will heighten sexual feeling while improving the muscle tone.

1 Draw up the muscles of the pelvic floor.
2 Hold for a count of two and then release. As you release, push very gently so that the vagina opens slightly.
3 Relax and repeat.

Once you feel that you are successfully mastering these muscles, progress to pulling the muscles up in **three stages,** holding at each stage. *Repeat* the process in reverse by slowly releasing the muscles once more in three stages. If you have stitches, you may feel them pulling as you release. Do not press down hard and do not hold your breath.

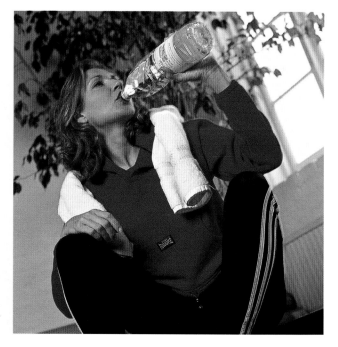

Rectus muscle distention

After delivery, most women will have a gap between the two muscles in the stomach, known as the rectus muscles. Sometimes they can separate. Normally after birth there is a gap of up to 2 fingers' width apart, or about 3 cm/1¼ inches. If the gap is greater – up to 5–6 cm/2–2½ inches – these muscles have distended.

Rectus muscle examination

1 Lie on a bed or on the floor with your knees bent and feet flat. Contract the stomach muscles and lift your head and shoulders up off the mattress or floor.
2 Place the fingers of your right hand just above the navel, with your left hand down by your side. You will feel the two edges of the rectus muscles contract at your fingertips. Should you find that you have a distended rectus, consult your midwife, health visitor or doctor who will be able to confirm this for you and show you how to perform the correct exercises. At first, you will need to take extra care in getting out of bed and maintaining correct posture.

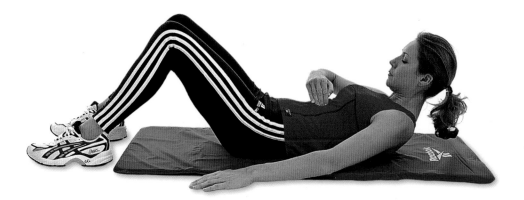

EXERCISE PROGRAMME FOR **DISTENDED RECTUS MUSCLES**

Abdominal retraction (see page 36) is the first exercise you need to do if you have a distended rectus. You can then follow on with **pelvic-tilting** (see page 36) and **easy curl-ups** (see page 37) from a supported position.

Pelvic tilting from a supported position
1 Rest your head on two pillows and cross your hands over the abdomen.
2 As you tighten the stomach muscles, tilt the pelvis and lift the head. Using your hands, pull the opposing stomach muscles towards each other.
3 Hold the position for a count of five, then lower back to the starting position. The breath must be used in conjunction with the exercise – **exhale** as you lift and **inhale** when you release the muscles. You must always tighten the stomach muscles before you lift the head and shoulders.

Once the gap between the rectus muscles has reduced to 3 cm/1¼ inches, you can add the **other abdominal exercises** (see pages 37, 42–43 and 56) to your routine.

Abdominal retraction

This exercise can be performed as soon as possible after birth, once you have tested for rectus distension.

1 Lie on your back with the knees bent, or sit down.
2 Pull in your abdominals and **hold** for a count of five. **Inhale** as you pull the muscles in and **hold** them.
3 Release the muscles while **exhaling**.

This exercise can be performed standing.

1 Pull in the abdominals and **hold** for a count of 5.
2 Release the muscles.

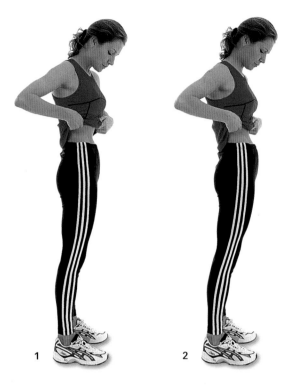

1   2

Pelvic tilting

1 Lie on your back with knees bent and hip-width apart, and the feet flat on the floor.
2 Push the lower back into the floor.
3 Tighten the abdominals.
4 Squeeze and lift the buttock muscles, tilting the pelvis upwards.
5 **Hold** for a count of five.
6 Release back down to the starting position.
7 *Repeat* this exercise eight times.

NB: This exercise can also be done while standing.

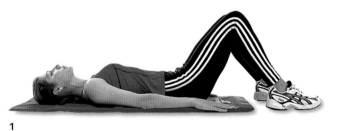

1

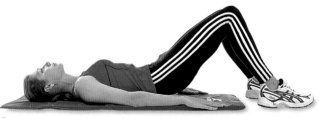

2

Oblique curl-ups

1 Lie on your back with knees bent and hip-width apart, and the lower back pushed into the floor.
2 **Exhale** and lift your shoulders, head and neck, but keep your chin tucked towards your chest.
3 Slide your left hand across to the right knee. The abdominals will contract as you push forwards and up. Keep your lower back firmly on the mat.

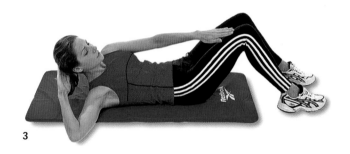

3

4 **Exhale** on the way up and **inhale** as you release and return to the starting position.
5 *Repeat with the right hand across to the left knee.*

6 *Repeat this exercise eight times* on each side, working up to 36 repetitions by the end of week seven.

Easy curl-ups

1 Lie on your back with knees bent and hip-width apart, and the lower back pushed into the floor.
2 **Exhale** and lift your shoulders. Slide your hands forward, keep the head and neck up, and your chin tucked in towards your chest.
3 Slide your hands towards your knees.
4 **Hold** for a count of four, release, then slide down to the starting position.
5 *Repeat this exercise eight times*, aiming to build up to three sets of eight curl-ups.

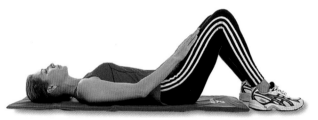

1

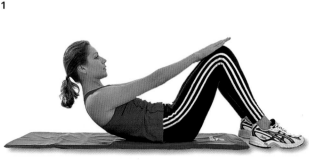

3

Ankle rotation

1 Lie on the bed or on the floor with the legs extended.
2 Lift and circle the right ankle five times anticlockwise, then five times clockwise.

3 Return the leg to the floor.
4 Lift and rotate the left ankle five times in each direction.

Warm-up exercises

These exercises will be part of your warm-up routine for the 10-week plan (see pages 84–125). **You need to carry them out before you move on to the other exercises so that the muscles of the body are warm.** The stretches are particularly important. You need to do these at the end as well as the beginning of your exercise session.

Shoulder shrugs

1 Lift your shoulders up to your ears and squeeze them together while you **inhale**.
2 Pull your shoulders down while **exhaling**.

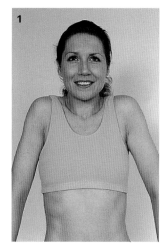
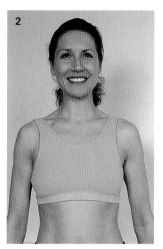

Shoulder rolls

1 Standing up straight with your shoulders relaxed, lift your shoulders up backwards and then forwards.
2 Circle this way for *eight lifts*, then change direction and circle for a further *eight lifts*.
3 Keep your shoulders relaxed, your neck long.

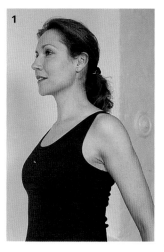

Head turns

1 Standing up straight with your shoulders relaxed, turn your head slowly to the left to look over your left shoulder, feeling the stretch on the side of your neck.
2 Return slowly to the central position.
3 Turn slowly to the right.
4 *Repeat* twice *each side*, moving at a slow pace. Keep your shoulders relaxed and check your posture.

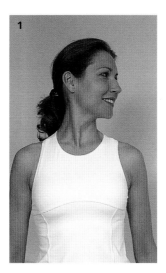

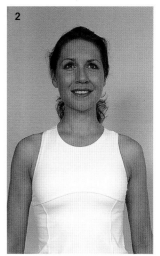

Neck stretch

1 Check your posture and **inhale**. Stand facing forwards with your feet slightly apart with your toes facing forwards and your arms hanging loosely at your sides.
2 Drop your head to one side, stretching hard downwards to try to touch your shoulder with your ear. **Exhale**. Ease out the tension by letting your neck stretch.
3 **Hold** for five seconds.
4 *Repeat on the other side.*

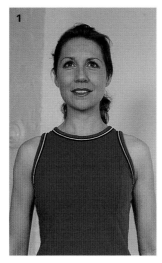

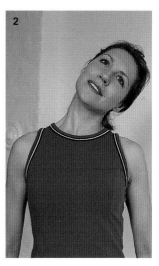

Shoulder stretch

1 Stand with your shoulders relaxed and arms hanging loosely at your sides.
2 Squeeze your shoulder blades back and together. Try to ensure that you do not lift them as you squeeze them.
3 **Hold** the position for a count of five before releasing.

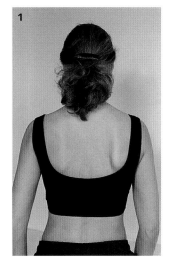
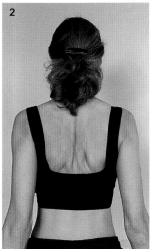

Side stretch

1 With feet hip-width apart, slide your right arm down your right leg, allowing your shoulders and your head to drop over to the right. Pull in your abdominals and feel the stretch down your side.
2 Stretch your fingers and **exhale**.
3 **Inhale** and come back up to the starting position.
4 *Repeat on the left-hand side*. You can build up this exercise, aiming for eight stretches each side. At first you may feel your side muscles pull and stretch considerably. **Do not bounce** while in this position.

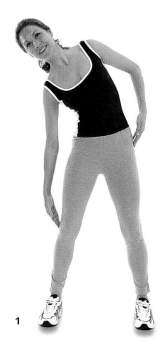

Side bends

1 With feet hip-width apart, stand with your arms hanging loosely at your sides.
2 Place your left hand on your hip and raise your right arm keeping your shoulders relaxed.
3 **Exhale** and stretch up and over to the left, feeling the stretch all the way up the right side of your body.
4 Return to the centre and *repeat on the other side*. Aim to do eight stretches on each side.

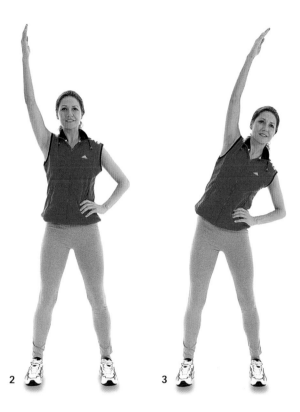

2

3

Leg swings

1 Stand up straight beside a windowsill with your left hand resting on it, or hold firmly on to the back of a chair with your left hand.
2 Keep your body straight. Lift your right leg and swing it forwards and backwards. Keep your knee bent and relaxed, with the movement coming from your hip. The idea is not to see how high you can lift your leg but to open the hip. You may find it easier to balance if you hold your right hand out just below shoulder level.
3 Do ten swings, then *repeat with your other leg*.

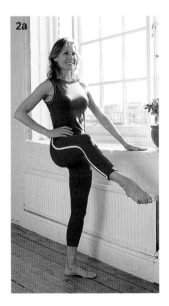

2a

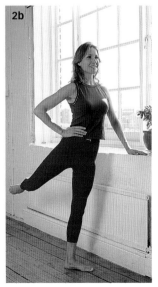

2b

Main exercises

These are the main exercises that will form the basis of the 10-week plan (see pages 84–125). **They must not in any circumstances be performed immediately after birth**, but can be started four weeks after the birth if no physical problems or worries are apparent.

Crunchies

This exercise is strenuous and you will need to build up to it.

1 Lie on your back on an exercise mat or towel with your knees bent and feet hip-width apart. Press your lower back into the floor to bring your pubic bone and pelvis up slightly.

2 Place your hands behind your head, with your elbows out to the side. There should be no strain through the neck, and the chin should be off the chest.

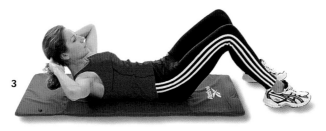

3

3 **Exhale** and lift up towards the ceiling, squeezing your abdominal muscles as you go. Keep your lower back on the mat, there should be no strain through your back.

4 **Inhale** as you release the abdominal muscles and return to the start position.

Curl downs

1 Sit with your knees bent and feet hip-width apart. Turn your toes in slightly and hold your arms out in front of you.

2 Slowly lower your back towards the floor, **exhaling** as you go. Be very careful not to overstretch.

3 Keep your chin near your chest and your shoulders relaxed. Squeeze your abdominals as you push yourself back up to the starting position.

4 *Repeat eight times*.

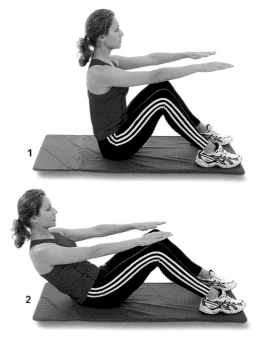

1

2

Extended obliques

1 Lie on your back on an exercise mat or towel, knees bent and hip-width apart.
2 Place your right ankle on your left knee. Place your hands behind your head, elbows out.
3 Lift up your head and shoulders and take your left elbow across to your right knee. Press your right knee back towards your elbow.
4 *Repeat before changing sides.*

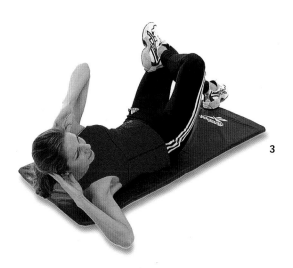

3

Small hip rolls

This is an excellent, simple two-in-one exercise for exercising the abdominal muscles at the same time as tightening the pelvic floor muscles.

1 Lie on your back on a mat or towel with knees bent and feet together.
2 Place your hands behind your head, elbows out.
3 **Inhale** and pull up your pelvic floor (see page 34) while squeezing your abdominal muscles.
4 As you **exhale**, let your knees drop over halfway to the right. **Hold** them in this position and **inhale**.
5 **Exhale** and bring the legs back to the centre.
6 *Repeat to the left side, then repeat three times each side.*

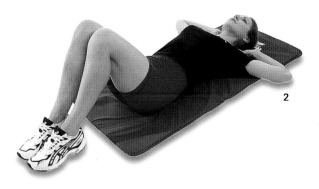

2

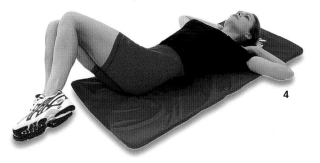

4

Buttock squeezes

1 Lie on your back on an exercise mat with your knees bent and hip-width apart.
2 Place your hands under the small of your back, lifting your buttocks up off the ground.
3 Squeeze your buttocks as you push your pubic bone upwards, pulling up the pelvic floor (see page 34).
4 Release the tension in the buttocks, but do not lower back to the floor.
5 *Tighten and release 12 times.* The buttocks feel as if they are being squeezed together.

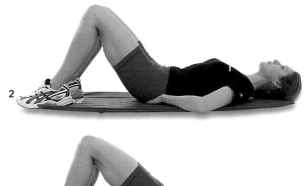

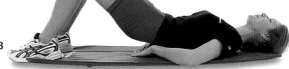

Cobra

This stretch will help to strengthen and stretch your back. Once you feel confident with this exercise and have performed it several times, you can progress to lifting the stretch further by pushing up with your hands as you lift up, straightening the arms so that the elbows come off the mat. The chest lifts up and you will feel a deep stretch in your back and through your abdominals. Keep your hips on the floor. Lower back to the mat as before.

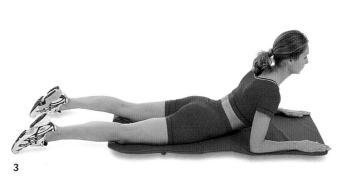

1 Lie on your stomach with your arms straight out in front of you, your elbows bent and hands flat on the floor.

2 **Inhale**, pull up your pelvic floor muscles (see page 34) and tighten your abdominals.
3 **Exhale** and lift your chest up from the floor but try to keep your elbows close to the ground. **Inhale**.

4 **Exhale** as you lower back to the ground. Control the movement and take your time so that you can feel your spine lengthening.

Doggies

This exercise will tone your thighs and strengthen your hip joints as well as increasing mobility within the joints.

1 Kneel on all fours, knees hip-width apart. Relax your head and neck.
2 Lift your right knee out to the side, keeping your heel lower than your knee. Pull up your back and abdominal muscles.
3 Lower your knee without letting it touch the ground.

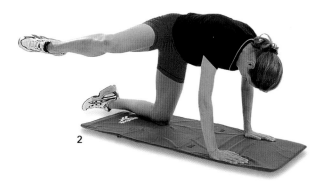

2

4 *Repeat the exercise eight times on the right and then eight times on the left.*

Pliés

This exercise shapes the inner thigh.

1 Stand holding on to a windowsill or the back of a chair with your feet pointing out and slightly wider than hip-width apart (the hip is rotated slightly).
2 Pull up the abdominals and relax the shoulders.

3 Keeping your back straight, **exhale** and bend down through the middle until you feel a stretch through the inside of your thighs.
4 **Hold** for a count of two before coming back up, **inhaling** as you go.
5 *Repeat eight times.*

Inner thigh toner

1 Lie on your right side on your right elbow.
2 Place your left leg on an exercise mat or towel, with your knee bent, and lift your right leg which is underneath you.
3 Lift and squeeze your inner thigh muscle. Turn your toes towards your nose to contract the muscle.
4 Lift your inner thigh up and down but without letting your leg rest back on the mat until you have completed *eight repetitions. Repeat on the other side.*

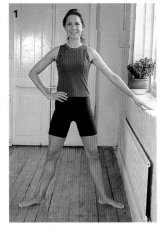

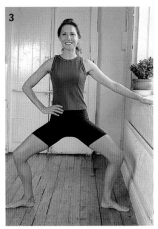

Leg lifts

This exercise tones the outer thigh.

1 Lie on your left side with your left leg bent and your right leg straight and raised off the floor. Rest on your left elbow with your right hand on the floor in front of you.
2 Keeping your hips facing downwards and turning your toes towards your nose, lift your right leg, contracting the

muscle along the thigh. Lower your leg to the starting position without touching the floor.

3 *Repeat the exercise eight times on the left then eight times on the right side.*

Easy press-ups

To begin with, you will need to work on easy press-ups.

1 Kneel on an exercise mat or towel on all fours with your palms on the floor, arms straight down from your shoulders and fingers facing forwards.
2 Cross your ankles and allow your hips to drop forwards.

3 Bend your elbows so that you dip your chest towards the floor, **inhaling** as you lower yourself.
4 **Exhale** as you push back up to your starting position.
5 Aim to do eight kneeling press-ups to start with.

Full press-ups

Once you feel comfortable with the easy press-ups, move on to full press-ups.

1 Extend your legs, resting on your toes, and keep your arms underneath your shoulders. Lower your chest to the ground by bending your elbows; at the same time lowering your hips.
2 **Hold** your abdominals in and make sure that your chest does not touch the floor.
3 Push back up to the starting position. **Inhale** as you lower and **exhale** as you rise. You will not be able to do many at first, but with practice you will be able to perform more. Alternate full press-ups with kneeling press-ups to build up strength.

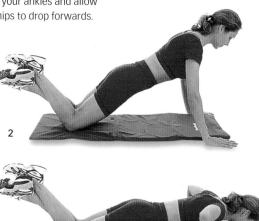

Biceps curls

1 Hold a small weight (you can use a small full tin of food if you do not have dumb-bells) in each hand. Standing up straight, extend your arms down in front of your body on your thighs, palms up. Make a fist with each hand.

2 Lift your arms straight up in front of your body towards your shoulders, squeezing the weights while bending your elbows to contract the muscles.

3 Relax and lower your arms to the starting position. *Repeat eight times.*

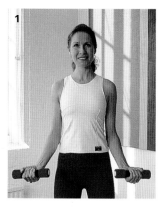

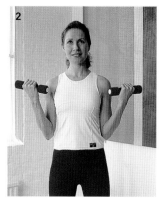

Overhead triceps curls

In order to take pressure off your back, this exercise can be performed in a seated position.

1 Hold a small weight in your left hand and lift your left arm straight up into the air.

2 Lower your forearm only, bending at the elbow, behind your head until the weight is between your shoulder blades. Use your right hand to support your upper arm if necessary. Straighten your arm slowly to the starting position.

3 *Repeat the exercise eight times on the left and then eight times on the right.*

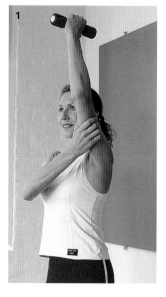

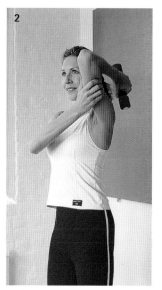

Triceps dips

As you become familiar with this exercise or to increase its intensity, lift your body off the mat or towel so that you support your weight on your hands. This works the triceps much harder, so do not attempt it until after at least two weeks of performing the exercise seated. With the feet firmly on the floor with the knees bent, bend your elbows and lower your bottom towards the floor but do not make contact. Press back upwards. **Inhale** on the way down and **exhale** on the way up. *Aim for three sets of eight.*

1 Sit on an exercise mat or towel with your knees bent and feet hip-width apart.

2 Place your hands behind your body and make sure that your fingers are facing towards your buttocks.
3 Relax your shoulders and bend your elbows, **inhaling** as you lower yourself down.
4 Using your whole body, return to an upright position, **exhaling** as you do so.

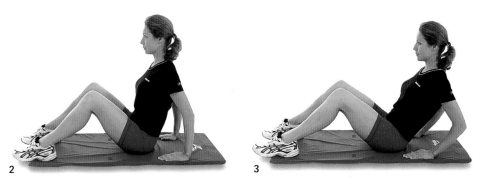

2   3

Weighted triceps

1 Stand with your feet hip-width apart and hold a small weight in each hand down by your sides or extend your arms out slightly backwards.
2 Bend your elbows and pull the weights forwards so that they come just below shoulder level. Keep your shoulders relaxed and do not bend backwards or forwards; only your arms should be working.
3 *Do three sets of eight repetitions.*

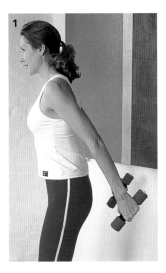

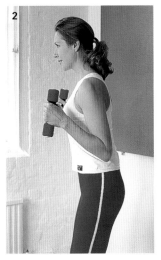

Roll-outs

1 With a small weight in each hand, lift your arms and stretch them out to the sides, so that they are held at shoulder height. Keep your shoulders relaxed.

2 Roll the weights back towards your shoulders by bending your elbows. **Exhale**. Squeeze the weights continuously, as this will make your muscles work harder.

3 **Inhale** as you roll the weights out again. Try not to let your shoulders or your neck area become tense.

4 *Do three sets of eight repetitions.*

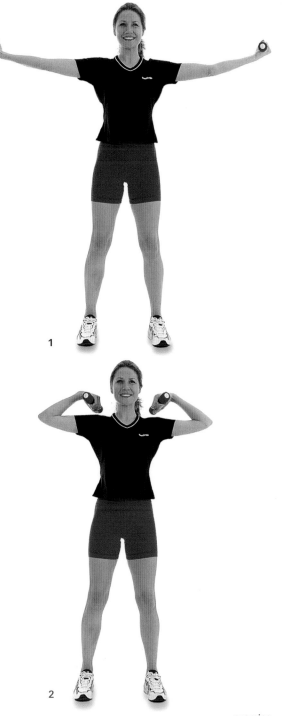

1

2

Thigh kickbacks

1 On all fours, rest forwards on your elbows.
2 Lift your right leg, bending at the knee. Pull up your abdominals and hold your foot flat, with the sole uppermost towards the ceiling.

3 Lift your right leg up, squeeze your buttocks at the same time. **Do not make a jerking movement**. Pull up your abdominal muscles and allow your head to drop forwards so that your back is not strained.

4 Return to the starting position, trying to keep your knee in line with your hip.
5 *Repeat eight times with your right leg and then eight times with your left leg.*

2

3

Lunges

These are quite powerful movements and will tone the thigh as well as increase strength in the leg and aid mobility in the hip.

1 Stand up straight with your feet hip-width apart. For balance, you may want to hold a small weight or a small full can in each hand.

2 Take a large step forwards on to your left leg, bending your knee. At the same time raise your forearms, palms up, into a horizontal position.

3 Bend your right knee at the same time, letting it drop towards the ground. Keep your front knee directly over your foot. **Inhale** as you bend down and raise your hands to your chest.

4 Using your left thigh, push back up and bring your left leg back to its starting position, **exhaling** as you do so.

5 *Repeat eight times on your left leg, then eight times on your right leg.* If you find the strain too great to begin with, you can use each leg alternately until you build up your leg muscles.

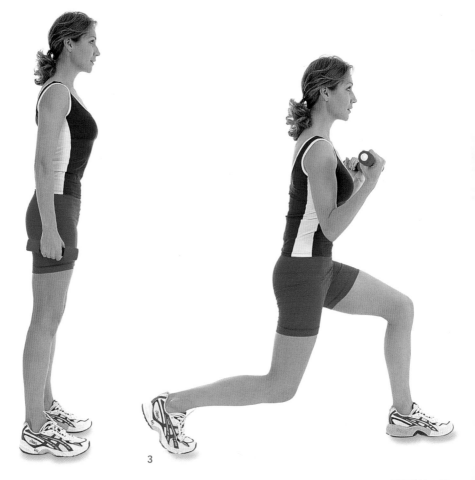

1

3

Waist-whittler

This exercise does just what its name suggests. Keep your back straight throughout the exercise.

1 Stand with your feet slightly further than hip-width apart. Pull in your abdominal muscles and keep your back straight.

2 Place your hands behind your head, elbows out, with your shoulders relaxed and pulled back.

3 With your hips facing forwards, twist slowly to the right.

4 Return back to the centre, then twist slowly to the left before returning to the centre.

5 *Repeat eight times on each side.*

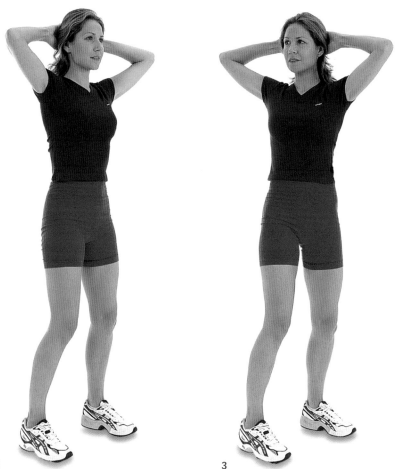

2

3

Cat stretch

This is a yoga posture that will stretch your spine, promoting strength and flexibility. It will also help release tension from your back and relieve backache. Make sure that you position an exercise mat or towel underneath your knees for this exercise. It should be carried out at a a slow pace with the maximum of control.

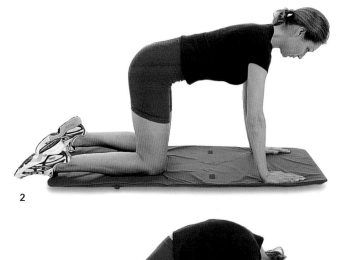

1 Kneel on all fours with your knees hip-width apart.

2 Flatten your back so that it is parallel to the floor and make sure that your head is in line with your back.

3 Pull up your stomach so that you arch your back, relaxing your head down and under while you **inhale**.

4 **Exhale** and release your back to counteract the stretch, pushing it towards the floor so that it is concave. Allow your head to come up and back.

5 Return to the starting position.

6 *Repeat four times.*

2

3

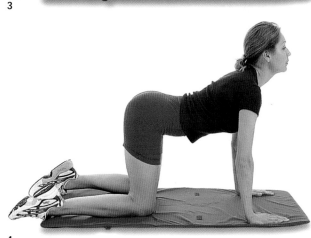

4

Hip flexor stretch

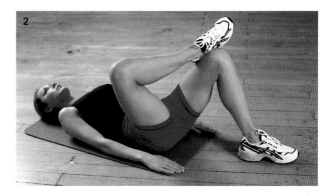

1 Lie on your back on an exercise mat or towel with your feet on the floor, knees bent.
2 Take hold of your right knee and pull it up on to your chest, then place your right ankle on your left knee. Relax your arms.
3 Slide your hands underneath your left thigh near the back of your knee and lift, pressing your right knee back and down. Feel the stretch in your buttocks and thighs.
4 *Repeat with your left leg.*

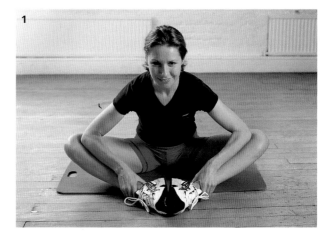

Inner thigh stretch

This exercise should be carried out slowly and with deep concentration.

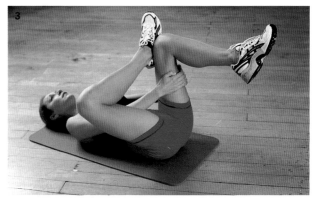

1 Sit on an exercise mat or towel, place the soles of your feet together and allow your knees to drop out towards the floor.
2 Lean slightly forward towards your heels and **exhale** as you feel the stretch through your inner thighs. Pull up your pelvic floor muscles.
3 **Hold** the position for a count of eight.
4 Bring your knees back together.

Hamstring stretch

1 Sit on the floor with your left leg stretched out in front of you and your back straight.

2 Place the sole of your right foot against the inner thigh of your left leg. Allow your right knee to drop out towards the floor. There should be no tension in your bent knee.

3 Stretch up with your body before lowering your chest forwards towards your left outstretched leg. **Exhale** as you go down. **Do not try to place your head on your knee** but reach towards your shin with your chest.

4 **Hold** for a count of five.

5 **Inhale** as you return to the upright position.

6 *Repeat the exercise on this side before changing legs.*

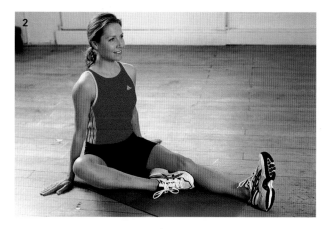

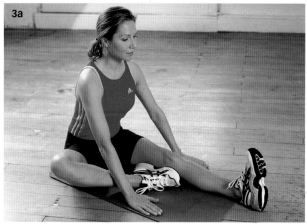

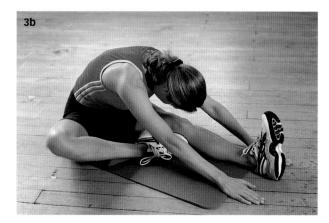

Exercises with your baby

Once you start on an exercise programme, you will notice that your strength and stamina quickly improve. Being unable to find time for exercise is one of the most common reasons why women give up. If you find that your baby is often awake and restless without you, then simply incorporate her into your routine. This will make it fun for both you and your baby. Obviously, you need to be aware of your limitations in terms of your strength. **Do not attempt to lift your baby over your head if you feel that she is too heavy or is struggling too much. It is inadvisable to exercise with your baby immediately after a feed.**

Abdominals

1 Lie on your back on an exercise mat or towel making sure that your lower back is in contact with the floor.
2 Sit your baby on your tummy, resting against your thighs.

3 Hold her under the armpits and lift your head and shoulders off the mat, **exhaling** as you lift up. You are now looking directly at your baby. Keep a gap between your chin and chest. Squeeze your abdominals as

you bring your chest towards the baby. You should be able to feel your stomach muscles contract as you lift.
4 Relax back and **inhale** as you return to the starting position.
5 *Work towards eight repetitions.*

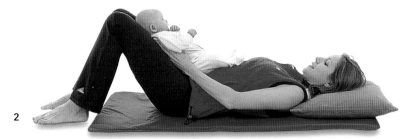

2

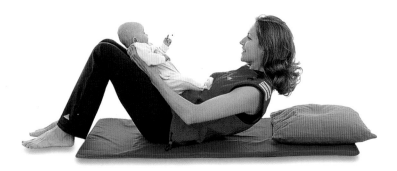

3

Upper-body toning

1 Cradle your baby comfortably on your lap facing you. Support her under the armpits and lie back. Make sure that you tip your pelvis gently up so that your lower back is on the floor and your knees are bent. Your feet should be hip-width apart.

2 **Inhale** and as you **exhale** lift your baby towards the ceiling. Keep your arms straight towards the ceiling and feel the push from your upper arms. Extend your arms to where it is comfortable and safe but do not lock the elbows. Be careful not to swing your baby in this position, or you may become unbalanced.

3 **Inhale** as you lower your baby back towards your lap.

4 *Work up to eight repetitions.* But do **be aware of the weight of your baby.**

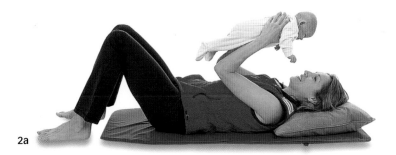

2a

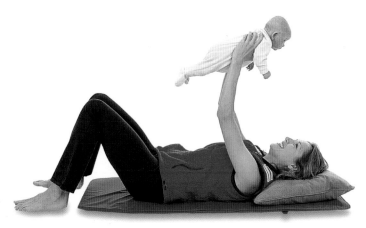

2b

Push-outs

1 Hold your baby under the armpits with her facing you.
2 Stand with feet hip-width apart. Relax your shoulders but check for good posture – your back should be straight and your stomach pulled in.
3 **Exhale** as you push your baby straight out in front of you, keeping your arms at shoulder level. This will work your upper arm and your pectoral muscles which support your bust from underneath.

4 **Inhale** as you pull your baby back towards you.
5 *Repeat the exercise, working up to eight repetitions.* Be aware all the time of your stomach muscles. The more you keep them tight, the better they will work. If at any time you feel that your baby is getting heavy, relax and place her gently down.

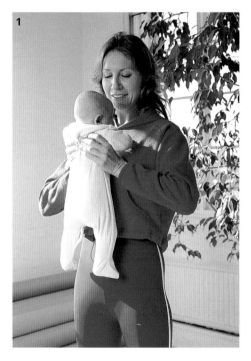

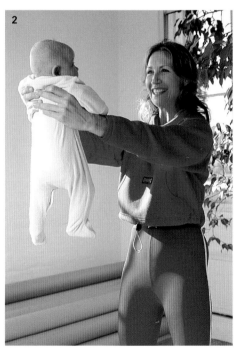

Leg lifts

This is a slow, thoughtful exercise that requires controlled breathing so that the muscles receive the oxygen they require. Once you feel comfortable with this exercise and you can lift each leg eight times, you can add a small bounce. Lift your leg and simply allow the leg to move up and down with a very small movement. Try this for eight mini lifts. Your baby may actively enjoy being bounced in this way.

1 Sit on an exercise mat or towel with your baby sitting on your left thigh, facing towards you. Hold her under the armpits and at the back of her head to support her. When you first try this exercise, it is advisable to have your back supported against a large cushion, wall or settee.

2 Pull in your stomach muscles, then lift your left leg by straightening your thigh and turning your toes towards your nose.

3 **Hold** this position. You will feel the tension through your thigh. At first, you will not be able to lift your leg far, but that is fine. It should never be lifted so that your weight is unevenly distributed by being thrown to one side. You will tone your leg providing your thigh is tightened.

4 Lower your leg and **exhale**.

5 *Repeat with your right leg.*

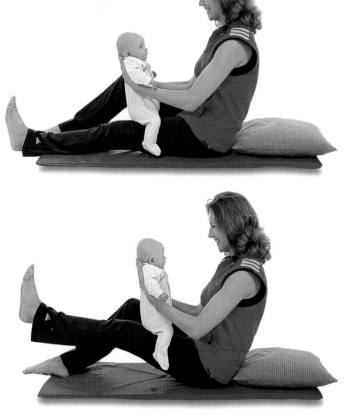

1

2

Wellbeing

Feeling good about yourself comes not only from what you look like on the outside but also how you feel on the inside. When you have a new baby and there is no routine to your day or night, and you feel that your entire world is chaotic and stressful, the thought of self-indulgent treatments may seem ridiculous. But when you feel better, you cope better.

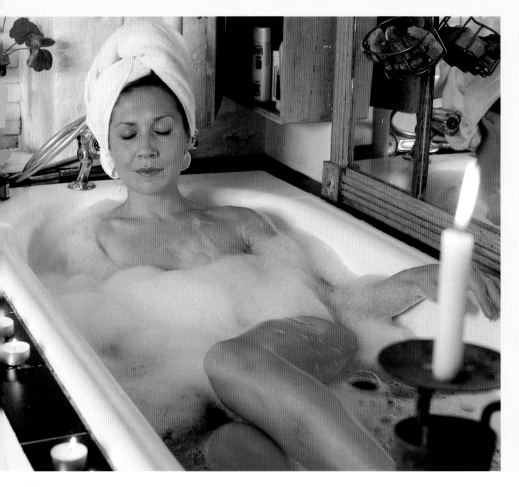

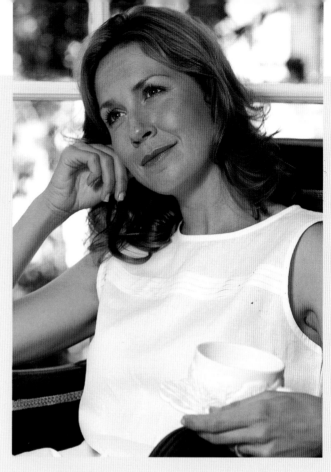

REBALANCING AND RESTORING

In becoming a mother, you add yet another role to a seemingly endless list – partner, wife, lover and carer. Thinking of finding time for yourself can seem impossible, selfish and an unnecessary extravagance, but it is actually vital. You have been through the biggest emotional and physical change ever, and consequently your body needs some attention to help it rebalance, restore and maintain wellbeing. The care and attention you give it will be reflected in your general state of health.

TREATING YOUR WHOLE SELF

The mind, body and spirit are closely linked, so that any attention to one area will have an effect on the other. Working on your body through exercise and diet may make you tone up and lose weight, but helping your skin to shine, your body to stretch and

Finding time for yourself can seem **impossible,** selfish and an unnecessary extravagance, but it is **vital**

your mind to relax will enable you to get the most out of life. Natural beauty treatments are soothing and restorative, while relaxation, yoga and meditation techniques will all increase your energy and revitalize you. In fact, 20 minutes' meditation is worth over one hour's sleep, which is probably by far your most important need at the moment.

HELPING YOURSELF TO COPE

After the birth of a baby, everything changes – your energy levels, your outlook and even your relationships with those around you, in addition to the physical changes that have taken place. Both looking and feeling good enhances your ability to deal with these new and exciting challenges in a positive way.

Strategies for enhancing wellbeing

For some women, finding the time to visit a health or beauty clinic can be just too difficult in the early stages of postnatal recovery. Self-help techniques and natural treatments prepared at home can be just as beneficial at a much lower cost.

FINDING TIME FOR RELAXATION

When your baby goes for a nap during the day, reserve this time for yourself. Breathing, meditation and relaxation techniques will help to restore your sense of equilibrium and replenish energy levels. For beauty treatments and massage, make an effort to create the right atmosphere in which to relax and enjoy to the full this precious time spent on yourself. Find a quiet room where you are most comfortable. Start with a warm bath scented by essential oils, or light scented candles or burn relaxing lavender oil in an oil burner. Soft, gentle music in the form of specially designed relaxation CDs or tapes can also be very soothing and therapeutic.

PAMPERING YOURSELF

Look for other, small ways in which to pamper yourself. Consider buying a new item of clothing or a whole outfit if you can. Rather than go shopping, it is often easier to order something from a catalogue or on the Internet. Buy something that fits you now rather than opting for a

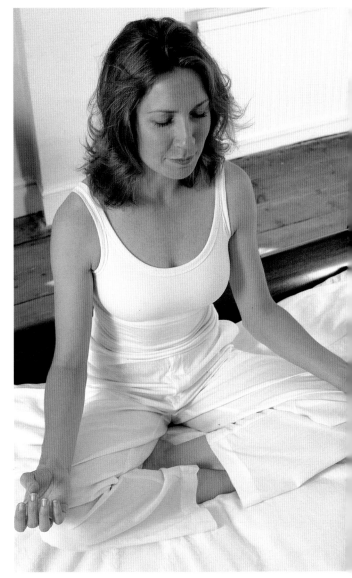

Breathing, meditation and **relaxation techniques** will help to restore your sense of **equilibrium** and **replenish** energy levels

size smaller with the aim of slimming into it. What you need is to look good now to boost your self-image and morale.

LIGHTENING THE LOAD

Many larger supermarkets in towns have a delivery service – it is worth paying a little extra for the shopping to be delivered, if you can afford it. Check this out on the Internet or phone your local supermarket for details.

Make a list of the jobs that you feel you ought to have done or be doing and prioritize them. This will help you to approach the tasks in a positive, systematic way and clear your mind of worry and burden. Consider whether you can get help with any of them.

ENJOYING THE GREAT OUTDOORS

Fresh air is very beneficial. Sitting in the garden for just five minutes will make you feel better. Go for a walk somewhere peaceful and attractive with your baby. A baby sling in preference to a pram or pushchair is ideal for walks across unlevelled terrain. If it is a sunny day, cover both of you in sunblock and enjoy it!

WELLBEING TIP

- Try to have some time to yourself every day.
- Don't forget to treat yourself.
- Make the most of the Internet and home delivery services to make your day easier.
- Accept offers of help from friends or family.
- Take some gentle exercise every day.
- Find a way to relax that works for you.

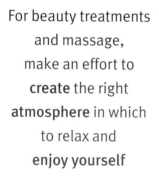

For beauty treatments and massage, make an effort to **create** the right **atmosphere** in which to relax and **enjoy yourself**

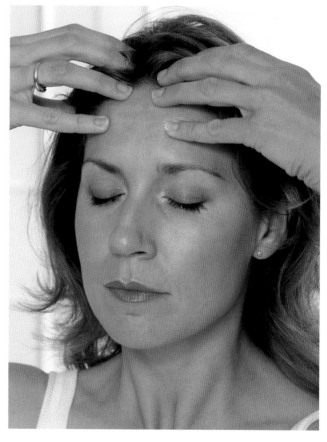

You and your partner

Having a baby affects both of you. Just as you experience mood swings, tears and feelings of anxiety, so can your partner. You have the excuse of fluctuating hormones; he does not. You have had the last nine months to consider the prospect of motherhood and experience the internal and external changes, while he has been a bystander.

Make an effort to spend time alone with your partner

UNDERSTANDING YOUR PARTNER'S NEEDS

After the initial euphoria of the birth has worn off, many men feel neglected and confused. Your partner's role, like yours, has changed. He will probably experience a range of emotions that he never knew existed – feelings that he may be too embarrassed to discuss. He may be just as bewildered by the whole event as you are and feel guilty about his needs.

You may want and expect your partner to take an active role in parenting, yet you may feel reluctant to hand your baby over to him. Many women scrutinize their partners as they take their turn in parenting. They can be quick to criticize or show them how to do it their way. Place your trust and respect in your partner's ability and recognize that although he may do things differently to you he is still capable. Fathers need their own space to be able to bond with their babies. Use the time he has with the baby to do something relaxing for yourself.

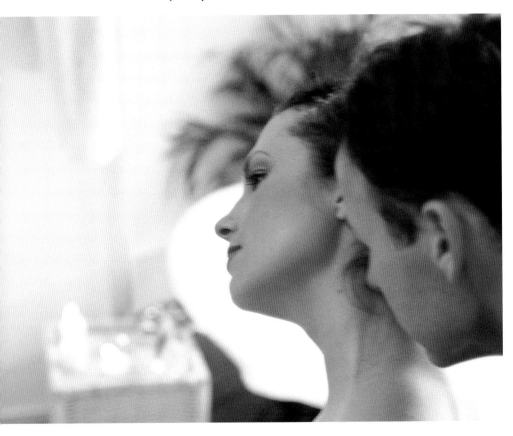

FINDING TIME TOGETHER

Making time for each other is the key. Your relationship and way of life was established in its particular way before the baby was born, and now there is much less time to spend on each other. Try to spend quality time together. A drive out with your baby in the car seat or a walk with your baby in the backpack may give you the opportunity to talk. Remember to listen as well as talk – we all feel supported and loved when we are listened to. Find someone to have the baby for an hour or two while you go out together as a couple for a meal, to the cinema or theatre, or simply for a walk. Getting out for a while will be beneficial to both of you.

Try to eat together whenever possible. If you find that you are very hungry while breast-feeding, try to plan your meal times accordingly. Otherwise, use weekends to enjoy dinner together. Do not be afraid to tell friends and other relatives that you are not available all the time; allow the answerphone to earn its keep by screening calls.

PAMPERING EACH OTHER

Include your partner in your beauty treatments and relaxation techniques. Giving him a back massage will demonstrate your feelings towards him, and he will be only too willing to reciprocate.

TALKING ABOUT SEX

Returning to sex cannot be determined on the basis of time; only you will know when it feels right to start again. While it is useful to have had sex before your

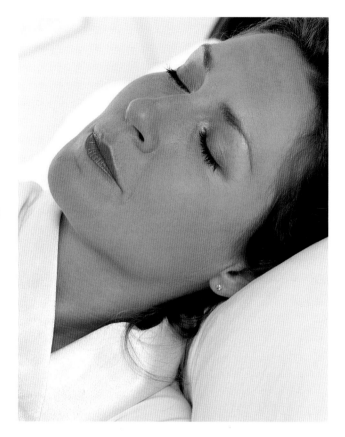

Going **back to bed** in the morning at the weekend can knock routine and boredom on the head, and **rekindle** your interest in lovemaking

six-week postnatal health check so that you can raise any problems with your doctor or health adviser, for some women this is unrealistic. Explaining your feelings and fears will help reassure your partner that you still find him attractive. Try cuddling, massaging and touching instead, and keep in mind that being loving and loved is the way in which you communicate with each other. If being overwhelmingly tired is the main cause of your abstinence, try changing the time that you make love. Going back to bed in the morning at the weekend can knock routine and boredom on the head, and help rekindle your interest in lovemaking.

Beauty treatments

Hair

After the birth of your baby, the change in your hair may be quite dramatic because of fluctuations in your hormones. It may suddenly become greasy, handfuls can fall out and it may have no lustre or shine. There is not much you can do about this except to be patient. It is perfectly normal for your hair to respond in this way.

A healthy diet, high in fresh vegetables, fruit, proteins, carbohydrates and some fats, will ensure that your hair is not deprived of the minerals and vitamins it needs.

RESTYLING

A visit to a hairdresser will do wonders for you, your hair and your self-esteem. Get someone else to look after your baby while you are there. The time spent away will help you to feel revived. If this is too difficult, consider contacting a mobile hairdresser or plan a home treatment. Consider how much time you have available for your hair. Long hair or a fussy hairstyle can be time-consuming to look after. A new style can be very rejuvenating. Let your hairdresser know that you have recently had a baby so that any changes going on in your hair can be accommodated.

COLOURING AND CONDITIONING

Adding colour to your hair may boost your self-esteem. Highlights will add colour to your complexion, giving an instant feel-good factor. A deep conditioner will certainly improve the texture of your hair.

HAIR **TREATMENT**

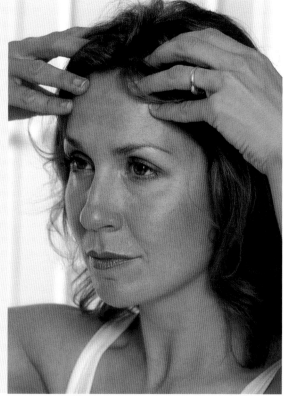

- A **scalp massage** will stimulate the blood supply to the hair follicles and so start feeding the hair and promoting thickness and shine. Pour a little sweet almond or extra-virgin olive oil into your palms and massage the scalp with circular movements. You can add lavender, rosemary, sage, cedarwood or ylang ylang essential oils to the base oil (4–5 drops to 1½ tablespoons base oil).

- Pay particular attention to the **top** and **the back of your head**, since this is where most tension is held. Massage for 5 minutes, then wrap a towel around the hair and leave for a further 15–20 minutes. Then shampoo and rinse as normal.

- For an **oily scalp**, pre-wash with the juice of half a lemon or 1 tablespoon vinegar diluted in 600 ml/1 pint water. Leave for a few minutes, then wash with a mild shampoo.

Skin

Your skin will change after the birth. During pregnancy you may have found that your skin glowed, and if it had previously been oily, it may well have dried. The depletion of nutrients by the baby during pregnancy will have taken its toll, and the change in hormones means that extra oestrogen, which helps to condition the skin, will not be produced. Now you may find that your skin is too dry. Add to this lack of sleep, lack of exercise, too much caffeine and the problems really start to show.

The liver is the main organ responsible for removing toxins. It responds badly to anxiety, stress, frustration and anger. Try adding dandelion leaves, watercress or parsley to salads to cleanse it. Eating foods rich in magnesium, such as bananas, raisins, spinach, potatoes and asparagus will help.

FLUID INTAKE

The body needs water to keep the skin hydrated, and water is also vital in helping the liver and kidneys to eliminate toxins from the body. A cup of boiling water with the juice of half a lemon added at the start of the day not only helps the liver but also tones the skin. Use the inside of the lemon to soften and whiten the skin of your elbows. Replacing tea, coffee, chocolate and cola with water will not only make you feel better but will make a positive difference to your appearance. Try substituting a herbal tea for ordinary tea. Peppermint, fennel, nettle and chamomile all have therapeutic and soothing qualities.

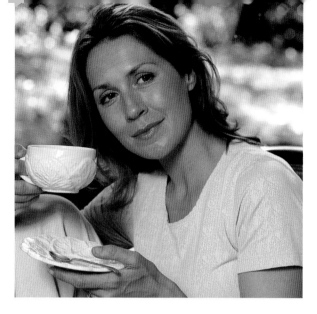

Making changes to your drinking habits can **rejuvenate your skin** and complexion, guarding against the **effects of ageing**

DIETARY NEEDS AND NUTRIENTS

Paying attention to your diet is very important at this stage to ensure that your skin has the capacity to re-tone and restore itself. It requires a variety of foods to ensure it receives all the necessary nutrients. Antioxidants (see page 21) are particularly beneficial to the skin, helping guard against free-radical damage that can make skin look old.

FOODS THAT DAMAGE THE SKIN

The main culprits are:

Sugar increases the severity and frequency of any bacterial infection since the bacteria feed off the sugar.

Saturated fats make the skin less flexible, blocking the capillaries that carry nutrients to the skin and increase the risk of clogged pores for people prone to oily skin.

Fried, smoked and barbecued foods are low in antioxidants.

Salt draws the fluid out of the body cells, drying tissues and causing the body to become dehydrated.

Tea and coffee eliminate body fluid through the kidneys.

Alcohol does the same and also interferes with liver function, causing a build-up of toxins that is excreted through the skin.

Skin treatments

Cleansing, toning and moisturizing your skin will all add to a clear complexion and a healthy glow. While it is important to watch what you eat and drink, it is also important to consider what you apply to your skin. You can literally feed your face, adding nutrients and vitamins through a home-made face mask. In all cases, ensure that you cleanse the skin thoroughly beforehand.

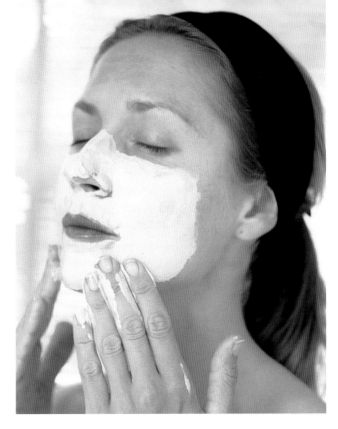

Refreshing toner

This recipe is for normal to dry skin. For normal to oily skin, use orangeflower water and bergamot and cypress essential oils. If using bergamot essential oil, avoid going outdoors for three hours afterwards, since it increases the skin's photosensitivity.

100 ml/3½ fl oz rosewater
1 drop lavender pure essential oil
1 drop frankincense pure essential oil

Mix the ingredients thoroughly by shaking them together in a small screw-top jar. Saturate a piece of cotton wool and dab lightly all over the face.

Avocado and honey nourishing facial mask

half an avocado
2 teaspoons live Greek yogurt
1 teaspoon runny honey
2 drops jasmine or rose otto pure essential oils

In a bowl, mash the avocado with a fork. Stir in the rest of the ingredients. Apply thickly to the face and leave in place for at least ten minutes. Wipe it off with a dry muslin cloth, then rinse the cloth in warm water and use it to remove the remainder of the mask.

Purifying face mask

2 tablespoons white kaolin powder
spring water
1 tablespoon fine oatmeal
1 teaspoon clear honey
sprig of fresh mint, chopped

Place the kaolin powder in a bowl and stir in enough spring water to make a paste. Stir in the oatmeal, honey and crushed mint. Apply to the face and leave for 15–20 minutes before washing off.

NUTRIENTS **ESSENTIAL FOR GOOD SKIN**

NUTRIENTS	WHAT IT DOES	WHERE TO FIND IT	EFFECT OF DEFICIENCY ON SKIN
Vitamin A	Antioxidant; helps to slow down the accumulation of keratin and keep the skin supple	Oily fish; offal; eggs; dairy foods	Scaly skin; flaky scalp; acne; poor wound healing
Betacarotene (pro-vitamin A)	Provides the body with the components to manufacture vitamin A; protects against the ageing effects of ultraviolet light and boosts immunity	Carrots; dark green vegetables; apricots; oranges; tomatoes; peppers; sweet potatoes; squash; pumpkin; watercress; cabbage	As for vitamin A
Bioflavonoids	Antioxidant; slows down the deterioration of connective tissue and strengthens the small capillaries that feed the skin	Pith and segments of citrus fruits; apricots; blackberries; cherries; rose hips; apples; buckwheat	Easy bruising; slow wound healing; premature ageing
Vitamin B2	Necessary for the development and repair of healthy skin tissue	Milk; eggs; cereals; liver; green leafy vegetables; mackerel; mushroom	Seborrhoeic dermatitis or inflammation around the nose and mouth; cracked lips; dull or oily hair
Vitamin B3	Helps the skin produce natural sunscreening substances, such as melanin	Brown rice; chicken; wheatgerm; tuna; broccoli	Dermatitis; acne; eczema; fatigue; depression
Vitamin B5 (pantothenic acid)	Necessary for the formation of new skin tissue to maintain healthy hair	Yeast; liver; kidney; eggs; brown rice; wholegrain cereals; lentils	Muscle tremors; cramps; fatigue; anxiety
Vitamin B6	Helps maintain normal oil balance in the skin and prevent allergic reactions	Chicken; yeast extract; broccoli; bananas; wheatgerm; beef	Overactive sebaceous glands, resulting in oily skin; flaky skin; water retention

NUTRIENTS **ESSENTIAL FOR GOOD SKIN**

NUTRIENTS	WHAT IT DOES	WHERE TO FIND IT	EFFECT OF DEFICIENCY ON SKIN
Biotin	Helps the body use essential fats; moderates the output of overactive sebaceous glands	Offal; wheatgerm; brewer's yeast	Dry skin, eczema; scaly dermatitis
Vitamin C	Antioxidant, so helps protect against free radicals; helps manufacture collagen; anti-bacterial, so helps to reduce infection on the skin; detoxifies, helping to eliminate waste	Blackcurrants; oranges; peppers; cherries; strawberries; broccoli; watercress	Broken thread veins; rough, scaly skin; easy bruising; red pimples; dry scalp
Vitamin E (tocopherol)	Helps prevent cell damage; strengthens blood vessels; maintains good circulation	Seeds; nuts; oily fish; sunflower oil; avocado; beans; wheatgerm	Premature wrinkles; pale skin; acne; easy bruising; slow wound healing
Folic acid	Slows down the loss of moisture from the skin	Brewer's yeast; liver; wheatgerm; molasses	Dry skin; eczema; cracked lips; pale complexion
Calcium	Helps skin regeneration; maintains good acid-alkaline balance	Milk; cheese; yogurt; almonds; parsley; brewer's yeast	Sallow, 'tired' skin
Magnesium	Works with calcium to build and slow down the age-related shrinkage that produces wrinkles; essential for muscle activity	Fresh green vegetables; raw wheatgerm; soya beans; milk; wholegrains; seafood; figs; apples; oily fish; nuts	Constipation, producing sallow and blemished skin; bone shrinkage; lack of energy

NUTRIENTS **ESSENTIAL FOR GOOD SKIN**

NUTRIENTS	WHAT IT DOES	WHERE TO FIND IT	EFFECT OF DEFICIENCY ON SKIN
Selenium	Antioxidant, so fights free radicals; helps body use vitamin E; reduces inflammation	Herrings; molasses; tuna; oysters; mushrooms	Dull complexion; dry skin
Silica	Needed for collagen manufacture	Horsetail (herb)	Premature wrinkles; eczema; psoriasis; acne; poor wound healing
Sulphur	FIghts bacterial infection to help keep skin clear; aids detoxification by stimulating bile secretion	Lean beef; dried beans; fish; eggs; cabbage	Dull complexion; skin infections; fatigue
Co-enzyme Q10	Supports immune system, so fights bacterial infection; antioxidant, so slows ageing caused by free radicals	Soya oils; sardines; mackerel; peanuts; pork	Depressed immunity; sallow skin
Zinc	Antioxidant; helps to make the protein that carries vitamin A to the skin; slows down the age-related weakening of collagen and elastin fibres; supports the immune system in destroying bacteria	Meat; wholegrains; brewer's yeast; wheatbran; wheatgerm; soy lecithin; beans	Dull complexion; eczema; acne; limp, dull hair; white marks on fingernails

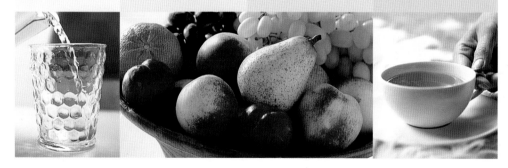

Bath treatments

Aromatherapy

Finding the time to relax in a warm (but not too hot) bath to which aromatherapy oils have been added can help to relax, stimulate or soothe you, depending upon the oils you choose.

Sensual bath

4 drops jasmine pure essential oil
4 drops ylang ylang pure essential oil
2 drops sandalwood pure essential oil

Soothing bath for aches and pains

4 drops chamomile pure essential oil
2 drops lavender pure essential oil
4 drops geranium pure essential oil

Relaxing bath

4 drops lavender pure essential oil
4 drops patchouli pure essential oil
2 drops rose pure essential oil

A home spa bath

This will help eliminate toxins from your skin and improve your metabolism.

1 handful of coarse sea salt
6 drops juniper pure essential oil
6 drops lemon pure essential oil
6 drops grapefruit pure essential oil
2 handfuls of dried seaweed powder or Epsom salts, tied up in a piece of muslin

Add the salt and essential oils to a hot bath. Use the muslin bag to massage your skin. Make sure that you keep the water topped up to maintain a regular temperature. Soak in the bath for at least 20 minutes, if not more. You may be surprised at just how hot you will feel.

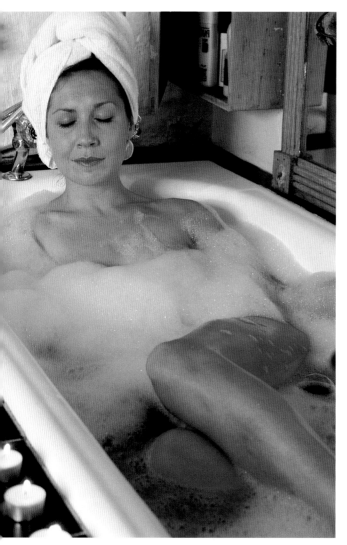

Refreshing bath gel

50 ml/2 fl oz unperfumed bath gel
10 drops bergamot pure essential oil
4 drops peppermint pure essential oil
6 drops juniper pure essential oil

Mix together thoroughly and add to the bath.

Body lotion

5 drops grapefruit pure essential oil
3 drops geranium pure essential oil
3 drops orange pure essential oil
3 drops ylang ylang pure essential oil
3 drops sandalwood pure essential oil
50 ml/2 fl oz unperfumed body lotion

Add the essential oils to the body lotion, stir well and apply.

Body scrubbing and brushing

Exfoliating the skin either with a homemade body scrub, such as bran and salt, or with a proprietary equivalent, will cleanse your skin and remove the dead cells. Dry body brushing is an invigorating and stimulating treatment that helps to smooth and soften skin. It stimulates the blood circulation, leaving the skin glowing, and boosts drainage of the lymphatic

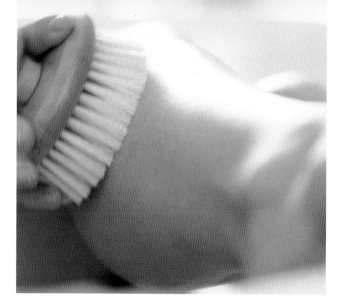

system, which helps eliminate toxins. A natural bristle body brush is best. Make movement upwards, and circle the stomach clockwise.

Try a body scrub before having a bath to cleanse, refine and soften the skin (see Refining Body Scrub below). After bathing, apply a good moisturizer to nourish the skin and leave it feeling soft and silky. If you have the space, position a few scented candles around the bath to aid relaxation.

Refining body scrub

1 handful of oatmeal
1 handful of coarse sea salt
4 drops grapefruit pure essential oil
4 drops lavender pure essential oil

Mix the oatmeal and sea salt together in a bowl. Add the essential oils and mix thoroughly. Rub over the body, then rinse off with warm water and pat dry. You can use a body brush to stimulate the skin.

Hydrotherapy

Hydrotherapy is another useful treatment and uses hot and cold water in the form of either baths or showers. The cold water restricts the blood capillaries while the heat encourages them to open. Water is well known for its therapeutic qualities. Spas, jacuzzis, whirlpools and foot baths all enhance wellbeing.

HYDROTHERAPY TREATMENT
This treatment is very beneficial to the lymphatic system and helps stimulate the circulation. Using the showerhead, spray yourself with warm water. Switch to cold only and using small, circling movements spray different areas of your body in turn. Pay particular attention to the thighs, hips and buttocks. Keep the cold water on for about 20 seconds before changing to warm for 1–2 minutes. Change back to cold. Dry yourself in a big towel and lie down for 10 minutes. Your skin will feel tingly and fresh.

Mind-body therapies

Breathing

Breathing properly is essential to our wellbeing, and is a widely respected and practised art in some cultures. While breathing is a natural process, it is easy to fall into bad habits. Poor breathing contributes to headaches, fatigue, insomnia and anxiety.

To improve your breathing, perform the Simple Breathing Exercise here. The key is to draw the breath into the lower ribcage.

Relaxation

Relaxation techniques can be used before meditation. You may find them more useful if you lie down. Muscle isolation – systematically tensing each muscle throughout the body – is the easiest method. The tension in the muscle heightens your awareness of it so that you can then feel when the muscle relaxes. Hold your breath when the muscles are contracted and release it when you release the muscles.

Visualization

Once you have learned how to relax, try a relaxation visualization. Shut your eyes and picture a place special to you that symbolizes security and stillness. Now sense the sun on your face, the birds and colours around you and the feeling of warmth from the sun. Make sure you are alone in this place and allow yourself to drift there for 10–20 minutes.

BREATHING EXERCISES

SIMPLE BREATHING EXERCISE
Use this exercise to focus on the process of breathing.

1 Stand or sit up straight.
2 Close your eyes and **focus on your breathing**.
3 Take a few slow, deep breaths and relax.
4 Visualize your lower ribs moving gently out on the **in-breath**.
5 Release the **out-breath**.

HEADACHE RELIEF
This breathing exercise should be performed slowly.

1 Raise the arms to shoulder height and place the fingertips of each hand on the forehead. **Inhale** and draw the fingertips of each hand across your forehead until they reach the temples.
2 As you **exhale**, stroke the fingertips slowly back to the centre of your forehead until they touch.
3 *Repeat the exercise until the pain fades.*

RELAXATION TECHNIQUE

1 Lie on your back, squeeze your toes as you **inhale** and **hold** the tension and **your breath for a count of five.**
2 **Release** the tension in the toes and **release the breath.**
3 Pull up your calf muscles and **hold for a count of five** while you **hold your in-breath.**
4 **Release** both the muscles and the breath.
5 Work your way up the body, focusing on each major muscle set in turn: buttocks, stomach, arms, hands, shoulders, head and facial muscles. **Hold each set for a count of five** before you release.

Meditation

This enhances the immune system and reduces blood pressure, while helping to focus and soothe the mind. Meditation is different from relaxing; it is a state of relaxed alertness. In other words, you are conscious of being focused on the sensations of the moment. It requires concentration and you may find that you have to practise in order to meditate effectively, but it is well worth the effort. In as little as 10–15 minutes, you will be revitalized and your energies replenished.

As well as lowering blood pressure, meditation has a beneficial effect upon sleep, helps recovery from fatigue, counteracts the effects of stress, aids breathing and relaxes the body as a whole – mind, body and spirit. Meditation will also improve your ability to concentrate.

The sitting position is considered to be the best for meditation as it allows the spine to be straight. This enhances breathing, allowing the free passage of oxygen in and out of the body. Deeper breathing into the abdomen allows tension and stress to be reduced and relaxes the internal organs.

MEDITATION TECHNIQUE

1 Close your eyes and **exhale** thoroughly.
2 **Inhale** through your nose and allow your abdomen to extend.
3 **Release the breath** and your abdomen.
4 As you continue breathing, consciously relax each part of the body – first the feet, then the calves and thighs, working your way up through your body.
5 Be aware of **your breath** but do not control it. If it feels unbalanced, so be it.
6 On every **out-breath**, count 'one', then on the next **out-breath** count 'two' until you reach ten. **Count only on the out-breath.**
7 Remain silent for a few minutes.
8 Tell yourself that you are now returning to everyday awareness.
9 Feel relaxed and at peace.
10 Open your eyes and shake your limbs or stretch.

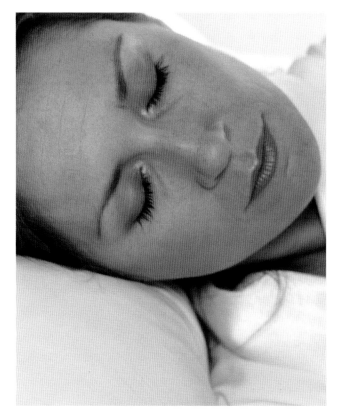

Meditation has a **beneficial** effect upon sleep patterns, helps recovery from fatigue and **counteracts** the effects of **stress**

Yoga exercise

Yoga strengthens, stretches and tones the muscles at the same time as giving mental relaxation. This yoga exercise will bring you renewed energy. Try to do it either outdoors or facing a window for light.

Salute to the sun

1 Stand up straight, feet hip-width apart with the palms of your hands together. **Inhale**.
2 **Exhale** and as you do so circle your arms up to the ceiling.
3 **Inhale** again, then breathe out and drop forwards, keeping your legs straight for as long as you can. Place your hands flat on the floor.
4 **Inhale**, then **exhale**, stretching your left leg out behind you. Your right leg should remain bent, and your hands should still be flat on the floor.
5 **Inhale**, then **exhale** and take your right leg back to join your left one.
6 **Inhale**, then **exhale** as you lower your body towards the floor by bending your knees. Allow your chest and chin to come into contact with the floor before your stomach.
7 **Inhale** and lift your chest from the floor, pushing up from your arms.

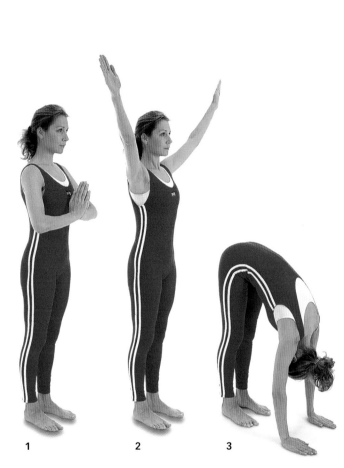

1   **2**   **3**

8 **Exhale** and lift your body up from the floor. Keep your hands on the floor and your head lifted.
9 **Inhale** and bring your left foot in under your left shoulder. Your right knee and leg are still lying on the floor.

10 **Exhale** and bring both legs together so that you are now standing, hands on floor.
11 **Inhale** and raise your arms over your head, then bend back to arch your spine.
12 **Exhale** and lower your arms to their starting position.

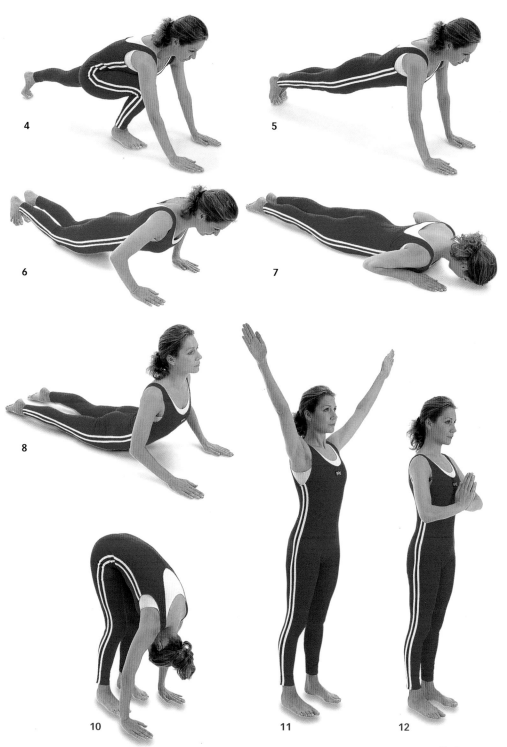

4

5

6

7

8

10

11

12

Massage

Massage promotes a feeling of wellbeing as well as reducing blood pressure and lowering the heart rate. It aids drainage of the lymphatic system, thereby helping to eliminate toxins from the body, and stimulates the circulation. The therapeutic qualities of touch are now widely recognized; massage is both relaxing and bonding. Getting your partner involved in massage will not only deal with any physical aches and pains, such as backache and shoulder tensions, but will reassert the emotional bond between you.

Since massage affects the nerves as well as the muscles, your stress levels will reduce. At a time when you may feel that any structure to your day has been swept away to be replaced with relentless and limitless demands on your time and energy, massage will restore vital energy and boost your self-esteem.

MASSAGE TECHNIQUE

In basic terms, massage is about stroking the body. Direct the strokes towards the heart, since this aids circulation. Long, flowing movements are soothing and relaxing. The whole of the hand is used with gentle, even pressure. A simple massage to learn and start with is a back massage (see opposite). Practise this on your partner and get him to do the same to you.

You need to create the right atmosphere to reap the full benefits of massage. Choose somewhere warm and comfortable to relax. Take the phone off the hook and play soft, relaxing music. Keep the lighting low and soft. Cover the parts of the body that you are not massaging with towels or a blanket, since massage reduces body temperature and you cannot relax when cold.

MASSAGE OILS

Oil is used for massage to allow the hands to move freely over the body without stretching or pulling the skin. It is usually a nut or vegetable oil, such as sweet almond, grapeseed, apricot or peach. Essential oils can be added to these base oils to enhance the effect of the massage. As well as creating certain moods, essential oils have a wide range of therapeutic qualities. Pure essential oils must always be diluted with a base oil before you use them. Massage oil should always be warmed in the hands before it is applied.

Relaxation massage oil

2 teaspoons diluted bergamot essential oil
5 drops mandarin pure essential oil
2 drops patchouli pure essential oil
1½ tablespoons grapeseed or sweet almond oil

Add the essential oils to the carrier oil and mix well.

Safety note: After bergamot oil has been applied, avoid going outdoors for three hours, since it increases the skin's photosensitivity.

Sensual massage oil

This will boost your sexuality and confidence.

2 teaspoons diluted bergamot essential oil
4 drops of palmarosa pure essential oil
2 drops ylang ylang pure essential oil
2 drops frankincense pure essential oil
1½ tablespoons grapeseed or sweet almond oil

Add the essential oils to the carrier oil and mix well.

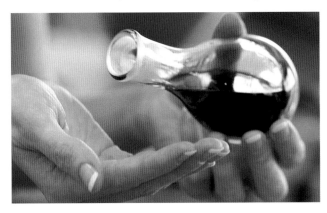

Back massage

The back is the most important part of the body for massage, and any massage to the back will have an immediate and powerful effect on the individual's entire body because of the high number of nerve endings present. Never massage directly on the spine.

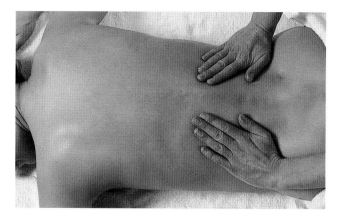

1 Pour a small amount of oil into your hands and rub between them. Place your hands together on the upper back and glide them firmly and slowly down the back, keeping the hands relaxed. Make sure there is equal pressure from the whole of your palms.

2 When you reach the lower back, sweep each hand out towards the hips. Bring your hands back up each side of the body simultaneously, keeping your fingers in contact with the skin as much as possible. This stroke can be applied more lightly.

3 When you reach the upper back, sweep your hands around the contours of the shoulders, and draw your hands together to meet at the neck. *Repeat the sequence two or three more times.*

Facial massage

1 Begin by thoroughly cleansing your face. Cover your face and throat with a thin layer of light moisturizer.
2 Place your hands at your jawline so that your middle fingers are resting on your jaw, just below your ears. Making small circles with the middle fingers, work your way round gradually to the centre of your chin. Keep your jaw relaxed while you do this. *Repeat three times.*
3 Return to the starting position, as in Step 2, but now make gentle pinching movements along the length of the jawline. *Repeat five times.*

4 To release tension in the forehead, place your middle fingers between your eyebrows and make small circles as you work your way out along the eyebrows towards your temples. Repeat this five times. Each time begin a fraction higher up the forehead until you reach the hairline.
5 Hold your earlobes between your thumb and forefinger and gently rub the lobes. Now work your way along the outer edge of your ears, gently rubbing all the way until you reach the top. *Repeat five times.*

6 To stimulate the eye area, begin with each middle finger on the inner corner of each eyebrow. Now make little tapping movements as you go. Work your way along the eyebrow; follow the eye socket round, across the top of your cheekbone and up the sides of your nose. *Circle your eyes five times.*

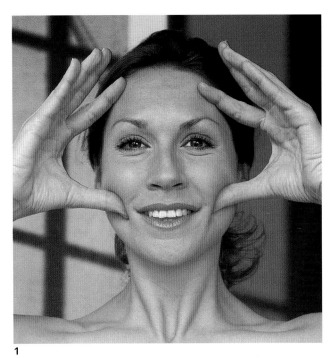

1

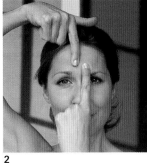

2

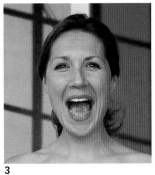

3

Unclench your face

1 Place your thumbs on your cheekbones and your index fingers on your forehead. Start at 12 o'clock and work round. Use your fingers to gently widen the area above and below the eyes. *Repeat*, circling the eyes in the other direction.

2 Hold the index fingers on either side of the brow. Draw them apart to release tension. Make sure the fingers stay on the same spot. Move along to the next area of the brow and repeat until the entire brow is worked.

3 Make an 'O' shape with the mouth and smile. Feel your lips being pulled back.

Repeat eight times. This movement helps to eliminate lines around the mouth and the nose.

4 Place the index finger against the inside of the cheek in your mouth. Blow and make a pooping sound. Try not to make wrinkles on the upper lip while blowing. This tones the lower cheek and mouth.

5 Open your mouth and gently move the jaw from side to side several times. Extend the lower jaw forwards to form an underbite, then make an overbite by retracting the lower jaw and chin. Allow your lips to come together in a natural way.

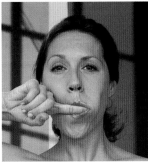

4

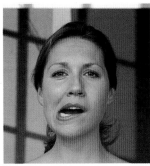

5

Abdomen massage

Abdomen massages can be done at any time during the day, maybe even in the bath if you feel comfortable. Massage can be started straight after the bath. Try to massage every day for the first week, then cut back gradually. Feeling the excess skin between your fingers may make you feel anxious about your weight, but as the weeks go by you will feel less and less of this skin.

Use sweet almond or extra-virgin olive oil as the massage oil, and remember to pour it into your hands to warm it before applying. Add lavender essential oil to the base oil for a soothing, relaxing massage, or use mandarin essential oil to help stretch marks to fade (use 4–5 drops essential oil to 1½ tablespoons carrier oil). If you find that you are constipated after birth, then massaging the abdomen should help bring relief.

1 Lie on your back or sit upright in a chair, whichever you feel is more comfortable.
2 Slide your hands across the abdomen from right to left, then left to right. Stroke in a clockwise direction, since this aids digestion.
3 Gently apply circular movements across the top of the abdomen, around the navel, around the hips and across in front of the pubic bone. Do not press down heavily.

Abdomen massage oil

2 teaspoons diluted chamomile essential oil
1 drop bergamot pure essential oil
1 drop marjoram pure essential oil
1½ tablespoons sweet almond or extra-virgin olive oil

Add the essential oils to the carrier oil and mix well.

Safety note: *Avoid going outdoors for three hours after using bergamot oil, as it increases the skin's photosensitivity.*

Anti-cellulite massage

You may find that with the added weight of pregnancy, cellulite has increased. Massage will help break down the toxins in the fat cells by stimulating the circulation.

1 Pour the massage oil into your hands to warm it.
2 Apply the oil and massage the thighs using squeezing movements, as if you are kneading bread, as well as sweeping movements. Massage upwards towards the heart.
3 Massage the hips, bottom and stomach in the same way.

Anti-cellulite massage oil

8 drops juniper pure essential oil
10 drops grapefruit pure essential oil
2 tablespoons sweet almond oil

Add the essential oils to the carrier oil and mix well.

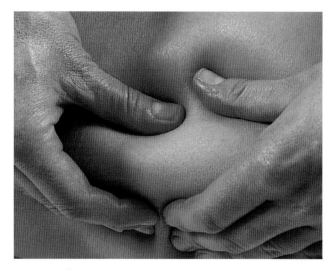

Foot massage

Generally one of the most neglected parts of the body, the feet play a vital role in health and wellbeing. The soles of the feet carry all the nerve endings and the reflex zones. A foot massage is very relaxing and pressing the soles of the feet at various points will help unblock different parts of the body.

1 Pour the massage oil into your hands and rub it between them.
2 Enclose the foot between both hands (one on top, one underneath). Slide your hands up the foot towards the ankle. This movement should be slow and soothing. *Repeat four times*.

3 Gently circle around the ankles using the middle finger.
4 Rub over the top of the foot with your thumbs in small circles. Work from the ankles to the toes. *Repeat four times*.
5 Rub each toe with the same movement.
6 Rotate each toe *twice in each direction*.
7 Gently pull each toe between finger and thumb.
8 Enclose the foot in both hands and rub in opposite directions. This is very warming.
9 Hold the foot firmly and rotate the ankle clockwise, then anticlockwise.
10 *Repeat Steps 1–9 with the other foot.*

Foot massage oil

1 teaspoon diluted lemongrass essential oil
1 drop geranium pure essential oil
2 drops sandalwood pure essential oil
1 teaspoon sweet almond oil

Blend the ingredients together and apply.

Revitalizing foot spa

1 handful of sea salt
4 drops peppermint pure essential oil
1 handful of fresh mint leaves, chopped

Place all the ingredients in a bowl and soak your feet for 10–15 minutes.

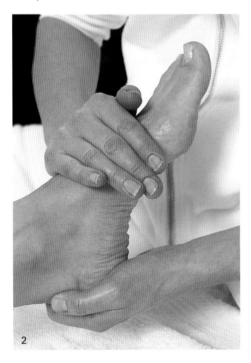

2

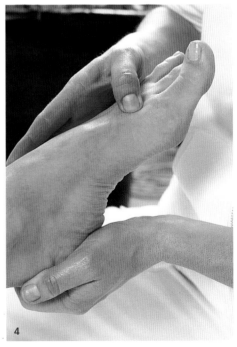

4

REFLEXOLOGY TECHNIQUE

Reflexology is based upon the theory that each area of the sole of the foot is connected to an organ or part of the body. The 'caterpillar walk' is a movement made by the thumb because it is stronger than the fingers. Use the outside part of your thumb – the part that touches the table when you lay your hands down flat. Bend and stretch the thumb as you wriggle it across the skin.

1 **Work the diaphragm**. Flex the toes of the right foot back slightly and apply pressure to the foot with the right thumb, just below the big toe joint. Use the caterpillar walk from one side of the foot over to the other.

2 **Work the spine**. Walk up the inside of the right foot with your right thumb, applying pressure all the way up. *Repeat three times*.

3 **Work the adrenal gland**. Supporting your right foot with your left hand, apply pressure about halfway down the foot just on the inside. Rotate the foot around the thumb as you press. Work the point for ten seconds and *repeat twice*.

4 **Work the neck**. Work across the base of the first three toes of your right foot with your right thumb. Now work across the top of the three toes where they join the foot, using either your left or right thumb.

5 **Work the shoulders**. Use the caterpillar walk below the fourth and fifth toes of your right foot. Work diagonally towards the outside edge of the foot.

6 *Repeat on the left foot.*

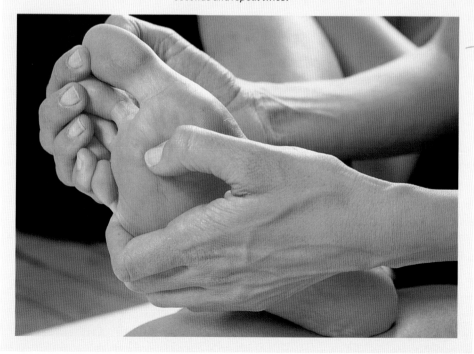

10-week plan

The 10-week recovery plan is designed to be easy to follow and to fit into your new life and changing routine. Taking regular, appropriate exercise, eating a healthy diet, and enhancing your wellbeing will help you to feel good about yourself and increase your energy levels.

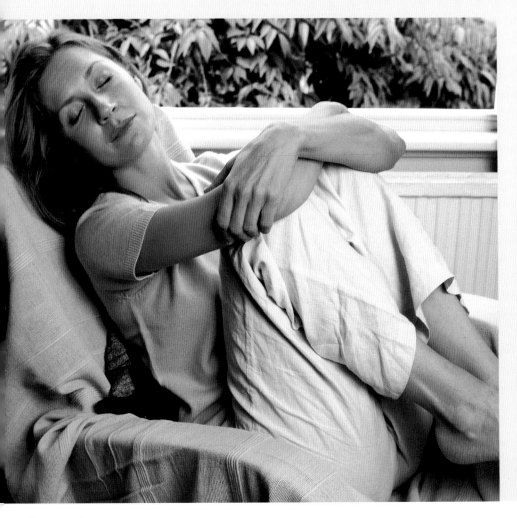

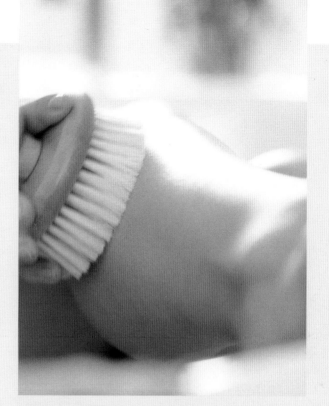

Welcome to the plan! You should be proud of yourself that you have decided to start this campaign to get yourself back in shape. Your recovery plan has been specially designed to be followed over a ten-week period, beginning four weeks after the birth. Starting the plan constitutes the birth of the new you, and as the weeks go by you will see how you have adjusted to having your baby, and how your healthy diet plan and exercise routine have gradually become part of your lifestyle.

NOTICING THE DIFFERENCE

The recovery plan is designed to be easy to follow and to fit into

Remember to be **kind to your body** – after all it has produced a wonderful **human** being

your new life and your changing routine. You will find that your energy levels rise and you feel better about yourself. Even if you have not necessarily lost much weight as such, you will notice the difference because you are fitter and your body is more toned. Should you find that you do not follow a particular week very well, you can always go back and repeat it. If for any reason you do give up halfway through the plan,

then simply restart it when you feel able to do so.

BE GENTLE ON YOURSELF

Remember to be kind to your body – after all it has produced a wonderful human being. Your hormones will still be in disarray at this stage, so try not to do too much or to have unrealistically high expectations. Remember that the key to good health is to look after yourself.

10-week plan

week
(1) 2 3 4 5 6 7 8 9 10

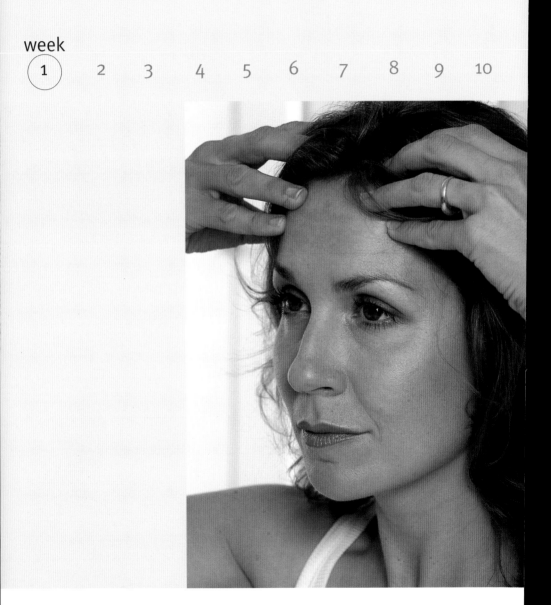

Week 1 planner

By the end of this week, you should feel a little more in touch with your body and have a different, more positive attitude towards it.

Exercise

The pelvic area is an important part of this week's exercise focus, to rediscover your muscles. Hopefully, you will have been doing your pelvic floor exercises (see page 34) since just after the birth, and by now the soreness and any stitches you had should have gone.

Now is a good time to think about going out with your baby for some air and exercise, but you must pay attention to your posture at this stage. Posture is important and using the Checking Your Posture exercise on page 31 will help you become aware of how you stand, sit and walk. Check that the handles of the pushchair or pram are high enough for you. Constant leaning over the handles will pull on your lower back, which will have been weakened through the pregnancy and birth. If you are using a baby sling to carry your baby, make sure that it is correctly fitted, otherwise it will pull on your neck and shoulders.

Diet

If you are breast-feeding you may find that you are incredibly hungry. Keep a supply of snacks available that release energy and top up your blood sugar but over a period of time – bananas or dried apricots, a handful of raisins or rice cakes. Cut up carrots, celery, cucumber and tomatoes and leave them covered in the refrigerator. A selection of fresh fruit is another healthy snack alternative.

It is also important to make sure that you are drinking enough. This will not only benefit your milk production but is also good for the skin, which may be excessively dry since the birth. Adding a slice of lemon to filtered or bottled water will add flavour. Try some of the many herbal teas you can buy or alternatively make your own (see page 16). Bear in mind, too, that if you eat hot and spicy food it may cause your baby to have digestive problems, so avoid anything highly flavoured in your diet at this stage.

WEEKLY PROGRESS CHART

Chart your progress on the 10-week recovery plan each week by making notes against these points. It will help you stay focused and motivated.

Date

Weight

How I feel about my appearance:

Skin

Hair

Weight loss

Muscle tone

Did I follow the diet plan this week?

Number of minutes/sets of exercises achieved this week

Monday

Breathing (see page 32) and **posture** (see page 31)	5 mins
Pelvic floor exercises (see page 34)	8 x 3 sets *3 times per day*
Warm-up (see pages 38–41)	5 mins
Abdominal retraction (see page 36)	8 x 3 sets

RELAXATION: **Aromatherapy bath** (see page 72).

TIP: When your baby sleeps during the day use this time to catch up on your own sleep. If you find it difficult to sleep, then rest with your feet up and read a newspaper or a book.

Tuesday

Breathing and **posture**	5 mins
Pelvic floor exercises	12 x 3 sets *3 times per day*
Warm-up	5 mins
Abdominal retraction	8 x 3 sets
Pelvic tilting (see page 36)	8 x 3 sets

AEROBIC EXERCISE: Take the baby out in the push chair or pram for 20 minutes' walking at a reasonable pace. You may feel slightly out of breath.
RELAXATION: **Unclench Your Face technique** (see page 80).

TIP: If you find sleeping difficult, give up tea, coffee, cola and hot chocolate at night, since they are high in caffeine.

Wednesday

Breathing and **posture**	5 mins
Pelvic floor exercises	12 x 3 sets *3 times per day*
Warm-up	5 mins
Abdominal retraction	8 x 3 sets
Pelvic tilting	8 x 3 sets
Pose of the Child yoga exercise (see page 93)	

RELAXATION: **Reflexology foot treatment** (see page 83).

TIP: Healthy food is what you require now, so make sure you have a bowl of raw vegetables and fruit chopped up in the refrigerator for you to dip into whenever the need occurs.

Thursday

Breathing and **posture**	5 mins
Warm-up	5 mins
Pelvic floor exercises	16 x 3 sets *3 times per day*
Pelvic tilting	8 x 3 sets
Cat stretch (see page 53)	
Buttock squeezes (see page 44)	8 x 3 sets
Hamstring stretch (see page 55)	1 stretch for each leg

AEROBIC EXERCISE: March briskly on the spot for 5 minutes, swinging your arms.
RELAXATION: **Unclench Your Face technique** (see page 80).

TIP: Try 20 minutes' walking with your baby, or without if you have someone to mind her. Relax those shoulders as you walk briskly. If you take your baby, use a pushchair or pram this week, rather than a sling.

Friday

Breathing and **posture**	5 mins
Warm-up	5 mins
Pelvic floor exercises	16 x 3 sets *3 times per day*
Pelvic tilting	12 x 3 sets
Abdominal retraction	12 x 3 sets
Small hip rolls (see page 43)	4
Cat stretch	
Buttock squeezes	8 x 3 sets

AEROBIC EXERCISE: 5 minutes' stair-climbing.
RELAXATION: Meditation (see pages 74–75).

TIP:Plan a week's menu in advance and get someone to shop for you this week.

Saturday

Breathing and **posture**	5 mins
Warm-up	5 mins
Pelvic floor exercises	16 x 3 sets *3 times per day*
Pelvic tilting	12 x 3 sets
Small hip rolls	4
Cat stretch	
Inner thigh toner (see page 45)	8

RELAXATION: Body brushing in the shower (see page 73) will help the skin and improve tone.

TIP:Calendula cream is soothing. Use it around the baby's umbilical cord if you feel that it is still sore. You can also use it to ease any stitches if they are still pulling.

Sunday

Breathing and **relaxation**	5 mins
Warm-up	5 mins
Pelvic floor exercises	16 x 3 sets *3 times per day*
Pelvic tilting	12 x 3 sets
Easy curl-ups (see page 37)	8 x 3 sets
Buttock squeezes	12 x 3 sets
Inner thigh toner	12 x 3 sets
Hamstring stretch	1 stretch for each leg

AEROBIC EXERCISE: Take a brisk 30-minute walk or an hour's leisurely stroll with your partner and baby. Let your partner carry the baby in a sling.
RELAXATION: Take time out for both you and your partner. Try to sit down together and find time to talk. Try a **foot massage** (see page 82) on each other with some peppermint essential oil diluted with a carrier oil. Burn lavender essential oil either in a burner or in the form of a scented candle and relax.

TIP: Divide your exercise into chunks. Three ten-minute bursts spaced throughout the day may be easier to achieve.

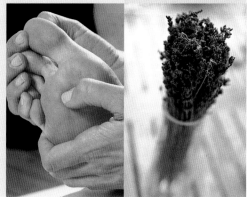

10-week plan

week

1   (2)   3   4   5   6   7   8   9   10

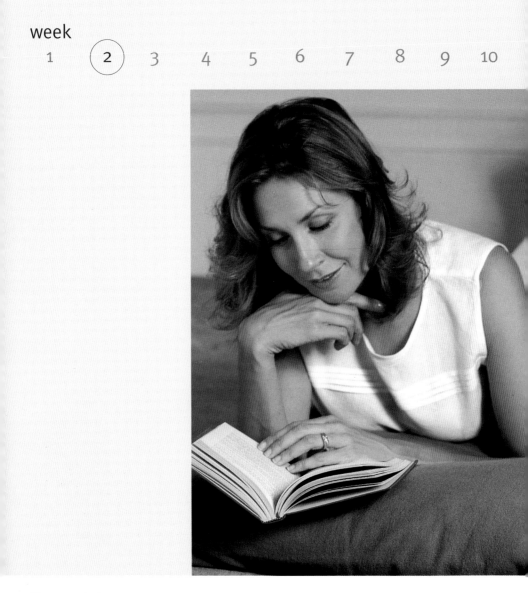

Week 2 planner

You began well last week, getting in touch with your abdominal muscles and starting to be able to control the pelvic floor again.

Exercise

You will notice that throughout the exercise plan your pelvic floor will be exercised. This is to get you into the habit of using these muscles. This week we will build on your stomach muscles, trying them out with some harder exercises. Remember to work at your own pace and make sure that you keep your lower back on the floor at all times. Do not forget to place a mat or towel on the floor before you do these exercises to protect your hips and knees. They are still vulnerable from pregnancy, so take particular care of them.

Diet

As the baby starts to feed for a longer period now, you are probably finding that you are not feeding quite so many times. If you are, do not worry; it will not be long before your baby settles down into a routine. Keep up your dairy intake to replenish calcium supplies and add a little extra fat. Now is not the time to get depressed – you are working steadily towards your goal of getting in shape. Try juicing this week to give you an instant energy boost, but be careful not to overdo it since juices are so effective at cleansing the system.

WEEKLY PROGRESS CHART

Chart your progress on the 10-week recovery plan each week by making notes against these points. It will help you stay focused and motivated.

Date _____

Weight _____

How I feel about my appearance:

Skin _____

Hair _____

Weight loss _____

Muscle tone _____

Did I follow the diet plan this week?

_____

_____

Number of minutes/sets of exercises achieved this week

_____

_____

week

1   **(2)**   3   4   5   6   7   8   9   10

Monday

Warm-up	5 mins
Pelvic floor exercises	5 mins
Easy curl-ups	8 x 3 sets
Leg lifts (see page 46)	8 x 3 sets
Inner thigh toner	12 x 3 sets
Small hip rolls	4
Inner thigh stretch (see page 54)	

RELAXATION: Try a treatment for your hair – **a scalp massage** (see page 66) will improve circulation to the area and help with any hair loss.

TIP: Are you on the Internet? If so, try some home shopping.

Tuesday

Warm-up	5 mins
Pelvic floor exercises	5 mins
Biceps curls (see page 47)	8 x 3 sets
Weighted triceps (weights optional – see page 48)	8 x 3 sets
Cat stretch	
Hamstring stretch	1 for each leg

AEROBIC EXERCISE: 7 minutes' marching on the spot; 5 minutes' step.
RELAXATION: Try a **simple meditation** to ease stress and rebalance your mind (see pages 74–75).

TIP: Buy your favourite magazine and read it from cover to cover.

Wednesday

Warm-up	5 mins
Pelvic floor exercises	5 mins
Pelvic tilting	12 x 3 sets
Easy curl-ups	12 x 3 sets
Doggies (see page 45)	8 x 3 sets
Cat stretch	

RELAXATION: Have an **anti-cellulite massage** for kick-starting those tough areas (see page 81).

TIP: Try drinking a cup of peppermint tea before you breast-feed if your baby has colic.

Thursday

Warm-up	5 mins
Pelvic floor exercises	5 mins
Biceps curls	8 x 3 sets
Weighted triceps (weights optional)	8 x 3 sets
Inner thigh toner	8 x 3 sets
Leg lifts	8 x 3 sets
Pliés (see page 45)	8 x 3 sets
Hamstring stretch	1 for each leg

AEROBIC EXERCISE: 5 minutes' stair-climbing; 5 minutes' step.
RELAXATION: Try a cup of rosemary tea – a sprig of the fresh herb infused for 5 minutes in a covered cup of boiling water, sweetened with honey. Add 8–9 drops rosemary essential oil to the bath in the morning. This will help energize you.

TIP: Find a relaxation tape of soothing music and play it in the early evening when you are feeding the baby

Friday

Warm-up	5 mins
Pelvic floor exercises	5 mins
Easy curl-ups	12 x 4 sets
Pelvic tilting	12 x 3 sets
Doggies	8 x 3 sets
Buttock squeezes	8 x 3 sets

RELAXATION: Burn frankincense essential oil in a burner while you use a visualization **relaxation technique** (see page 74).

TIP: Do not have too many visitors – it can be very tiring. Make sure you get time for yourself and your partner, so try to arrange for visitors to come in groups. When they have gone, put your feet up together.

Saturday

Warm-up	7 mins
Pelvic floor exercises	7 mins
Pliés	8 x 3 sets
Inner thigh toner	8 x 3 sets
Leg lifts	8 x 3 sets
Cat stretch	
Roll-outs (see page 49)	8 x 3 sets
Biceps curls	8 x 3 sets
Inner thigh stretch (see page 54)	

AEROBIC EXERCISE: 15 minutes' brisk walking or 30 minutes' gentle walking.
RELAXATION: **Hydrotherapy treatment** (see page 73).

TIP:Dim the lights, play some soft music and put candles on the dinner table, then order a takeaway.

Sunday

Warm-up	7 mins
Pelvic floor exercises	7 mins
Cobra (see page 44)	4
Small hip rolls	4
Waist-whittler (see page 52)	8 x 3 sets
Easy curl-ups	12 x 3 sets
Buttock squeezes	12 x 3 sets

TIP: Try a facial massage on each other tonight before going to bed (see page 79).

RELAXATION: **Pose of the Child yoga exercise** – kneel with the soles of your feet upwards and sit back with your back straight. Bend forwards to the ground and extend your arms in front, elbows bent. Open your knees to allow your tummy to drop though. Rest your forehead on the ground. Relax and breathe for 5 minutes, then return to the starting position.

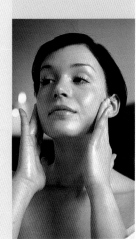

10-week plan

week

1   2   (3)   4   5   6   7   8   9   10

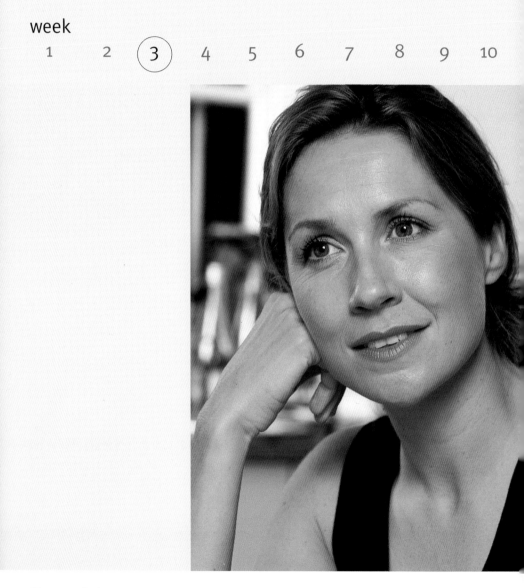

Week 3 planner

Breathing properly is very important, so make sure that you follow the correct technique (see page 32). Also, continue to check your posture throughout the day (see page 31).

Exercise

Pay particular attention to your stomach muscles as you contract them. The more you concentrate on them, the more efficiently you will work them. Remember that your pelvic floor muscles can be strengthened anytime, anywhere.

Diet

At around six-weeks, a baby's appetite often increases. If you are breast-feeding, make sure that your diet is full of nutritious food. Keep up your fruit and vegetable intake, and look for fresh seasonal produce. Try to buy organic food where possible. Bear in mind that you are less likely to snack if you are out and about, but do not skip meals or substitute meals with high-sugar snacks. Carry bananas or dried fruit in your bag, and if you feel the need to stop and eat, a baked potato is better for you than a fast-food hamburger.

6-WEEK POSTNATAL CHECK-UP

This is when you are probably going for your six-week check-up. Use this opportunity to raise any concerns or worries. It is advisable to have had intercourse before your health check, so that if you did feel any pain or discomfort you can discuss these with your practitioner. Expect your uterus to be felt to ensure that it is returning to normal.

Once everything has been found to be in good order, there is no excuse not to begin the exercise programme if you have delayed starting. So begin at Week 1 now (see page 88). If you had a Ceasarean delivery, this may also be a good time to start exercising.

WEEKLY PROGRESS CHART

Chart your progress on the 10-week recovery plan each week by making notes against these points. It will help you stay focused and motivated.

Date _____

Weight _____

How I feel about my appearance:

Skin _____

Hair _____

Weight loss _____

Muscle tone _____

Did I follow the diet plan this week?

_____

_____

Number of minutes/sets of exercises achieved this week

_____

_____

week

Monday

Warm-up	10 mins
Pelvic floor exercises	10 mins
Easy curl-ups	16 x 3 sets
Curl-downs (see page 42)	8 x 3 sets
Inner thigh toner	12 x 3 sets
Leg lifts	12 x 3 sets
Pliés	12 x 3 sets
Hamstring stretch	2 for each leg

AEROBIC EXERCISE: 10 minutes' marching on the spot with arms swinging;
5 minutes' step.
RELAXATION: Unclench Your Face technique (see page 80).

TIP: If your eyes are puffy from lack of sleep, try applying two cooled chamomile tea bags to restore and revive them.

Tuesday

Warm-up	10mins
Pelvic floor exercises	10 mins
Small hip rolls	4
Waist-whittler	8 x 3 sets
Cobra	
Salute to the Sun yoga pose (see page 76)	

RELAXATION: **Manicure your hands**. First, soak the nails in sweet almond oil, then file in one direction. Apply a nourishing hand cream afterwards. Mix up this massage oil for the hands – 1 teaspoon diluted palmarosa essential oil, 1 teaspoon sweet almond oil, 1 drop chamomile essential oil and 1 drop lavender essential oil. Mix together and rub over the hands and wrists.

TIP: Order a box of organic vegetables this week and get them delivered.

Wednesday

Warm-up	10 mins
Pelvic floor exercises	10 mins
Buttock squeezes	8 x 3 sets
Doggies	8 x 3 sets
Easy curl-ups	12 x 3 sets
Curl-downs	12 x 3 sets
Cat stretch	
Inner thigh stretch (see page 54)	

AEROBIC EXERCISE: 10 minutes' stair-climbing.
RELAXATION: 10 minutes' **breathing exercise** (see page 32).

TIP: Try this drink to leave you feeling mellow and relaxed – whizz up ½ mango, chopped, 1 banana, chopped, 150 ml/¼ pint apple juice and 1 teaspoon kava powder in a food processor or blender.

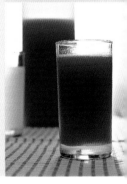

Thursday

Warm-up	10 mins
Pelvic floor exercises	10 mins
Weighted triceps (weights optional)	12 x 3 sets
Biceps curls	12 x 3 sets
Roll-outs	12 x 3 sets
Waist-whittler	8 x 3 sets
Cat stretch	
Pelvic-tilting	12 x 3 sets

RELAXATION: Place 2 tablespoons ground almonds, 1 tablespoon clear honey, 200 ml/7 fl oz organic milk, 2 drops patchouli essential oil blended with 2 teaspoons sweet almond oil, 3 drops ylang yang essential oil and 2 drops geranium essential oil in a food processor or blender and process until smooth. Run a bath and pour in the mixture. Soak for 20 minutes.

TIP: Try to exercise with someone else. This way you will make a commitment and stick to it. If you are trying a class for the first time, for instance, take along a friend. It helps get you over that 'first-time' reluctance.

Friday

Warm-up	10 mins
Pelvic floor exercises	10 mins
Curl-downs	12 x 3 sets
Easy curl-ups	12 x 3 sets
Oblique curl-ups (see page 37)	8 x 3 sets
Doggies	12 x 3 sets
Inner thigh stretch (see page 54)	

RELAXATION: Reflexology (see page 83).

TIP: Mothers may seem to interfere sometimes, but they can also have some good ideas. If you have the opportunity, talk your feelings and worries over with your mother and listen to what she has to say.

Saturday

Warm-up	10 mins
Pelvic floor exercises	10 mins
Small hip rolls	4
Inner thigh toner	12 x 3 sets
Leg lifts	12 x 3 sets
Plies	12 x 3 sets
Cat stretch	
Cobra	
Hamstring stretch	2 for each leg

AEROBIC EXERCISE: 15 minutes' marching or 30 minutes' brisk walking.
RELAXATION: Home Spa Bath (see page 72).

TIP: Check that your partner is getting exercise, too. It is no good you being fit if he is stressed and unhealthy. Encourage him into exercise – you could work out together.

Sunday

Warm-up & Pelvic floor exercises	10 mins of each
Curl-downs	12 x 3 sets
Easy curl-ups	12 x 3 sets
Oblique curl-ups	8 x 3 sets
Buttock squeezes	12 x 3 sets
Inner thigh toner	12 x 3 sets
Hip flexor stretch	each leg

AEROBIC EXERCISE: 1 hour's walking; 2 minutes' skipping; 5 minutes' stair-climbing.
RELAXATION: Meditation (see pages 74–75).

TIP: If you are on the phone a lot, use the time to do pliés to help tone your body.

10-week plan

week

1   2   3   (4)   5   6   7   8   9   10

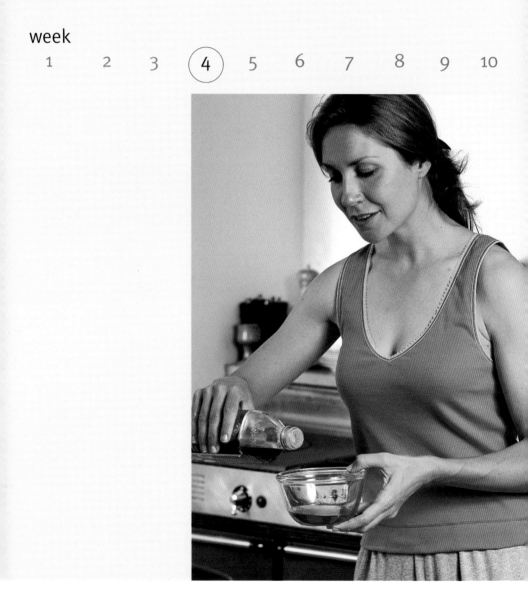

Week 4 planner

At this stage of the plan you are probably finding that a pattern is starting to emerge as to what time of day you are able to fit in your exercise programme.

Exercise

Your baby is probably quite happy, still in her bouncy chair, pram or cot where she is sleeping. If you find she is awake a little more, then keep her by you when you exercise. It is probably a good idea to put on some music as well. This will help to motivate you. Remember to wear loose clothes and a good-quality supporting bra. You should also wear something suitable on your feet now that you are increasing your aerobic work.

If you find that your pelvic floor is leaking a little, try to do some extra pelvic floor exercises during the day.

Diet

You may well be longing for something highly flavoured to eat, especially if you were careful during your pregnancy with herbs and spices. However, if you are breast-feeding, bear in mind that any spicy food may give your baby an upset stomach. However, if you feel a cold threatening, increase your intake of fresh garlic. This is particularly effective for fighting colds, and if the baby is suffering from sniffles, it will help build her immune system, too.

Try to vary your diet, and eat fresh fish when you have the opportunity. Make your meals quick and simple to avoid spending precious time in the kitchen. Stir-fries, risottos and pasta dishes are all quick and nutritious.

Chart your progress on the 10-week recovery plan each week by making notes against these points. It will help you stay focused and motivated.

Date _____

Weight _____

How I feel about my appearance:

Skin _____

Hair _____

Weight loss _____

Muscle tone _____

Did I follow the diet plan this week?

_____

_____

Number of minutes/sets of exercises achieved this week

_____

_____

Monday

Pelvic floor exercises	10 mins
Warm-up	10 mins
Waist-whittler	12 x 3 sets
Doggies	12 x 3 sets
Inner thigh toner	12 x 3 sets
Leg lifts	12 x 3 sets
Hamstring stretch	2 for each leg

RELAXATION: **Visualization meditation** (see page 74).

TIP: Take care as you lift your baby in and out of the car in her car seat to avoid straining your back.

Tuesday

Warm-up	10 mins
Pelvic floor exercises	10 mins
Curl-downs	12 x 3 sets
Easy curl-ups	12 x 3 sets
Oblique curl-ups	12 x 3 sets
Buttock squeezes	12 x 3 sets

AEROBIC EXERCISE: 10 minutes' marching; 5 minutes' stair-climbing.
RELAXATION: **Relaxation through muscle isolation** (see page 74).

TIP: Check the fat content of ready-made salad dressings. Instead, make your own with lemon juice and a little olive oil, adding herbs for flavour.

Wednesday

Warm-up	10 mins
Pelvic floor exercises	10 mins
Biceps curls	12 x 3 sets
Weighted triceps (weights optional)	12 x 3 sets
Roll-outs	12 x 3 sets
Waist-whittler	12 x 3 sets
Cat stretch	
Inner thigh stretch	

RELAXATION: **Reflexology foot treatment** (see page 83).

TIP: Phone your dentist! Dental care is free while you are pregnant and for a period afterwards. Your teeth may have suffered during pregnancy, so get them checked now.

Thursday

Warm-up	10 mins
Pelvic floor exercises	10 mins
Cobra	
Small hip rolls	4
Buttock squeezes	12 x 3 sets
Inner thigh stretch	

AEROBIC EXERCISE: 5 minutes' marching; 5 minutes' stair-climbing; 5 minutes' step.
RELAXATION: **Abdomen massage** (see page 81).

TIP: Contact your local leisure centre to find out about postnatal classes and crèche details.

Friday

Warm-up	10 mins
Pelvic floor exercises	10 mins
Leg lifts	12 x 3 sets
Pliés	12 x 3 sets
Inner thigh stretch	
Waist-whittler	12 x 3 sets
Hamstring stretch	2 for each leg

RELAXATION: **Back massage** for you and your partner (see page 79).

TIP: Resolve to drink three glasses of water every day from now on. Drink at least one before you exercise and one afterwards.

Saturday

Warm-up	10 mins
Pelvic floor exercises	10 mins
Easy curl-ups	12 x 3 sets
Curl-downs	12 x 3 sets
Oblique curl-ups	12 x 3 sets
Pelvic-tilting	12 x 3 sets
Buttock squeezes	12 x 3 sets
Hip flexor	1 for each leg

AEROBIC EXERCISE: 30 minutes' brisk walking with arms swinging.
RELAXATION: **Home Spa Bath** (see page 72).

TIP: Prioritize your week! Make a list of all the things that have to be done and that way you will be able to sort them into a plan of action.

Sunday

Warm-up	10 mins
Pelvic floor exercises	10 mins
Breathing and posture	5 mins
Abdominal retractions	24

RELAXATION: **Face cleanse, tone** and **feed** (see pages 67–68).

TIP: Strengthen feet and promote relaxation by rolling them over a wooden rolling pin. Make the movement from the toes to the heel.

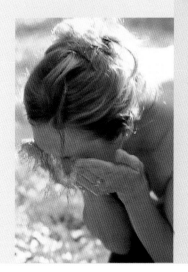

10-week plan

week

1   2   3   4   (5)   6   7   8   9   10

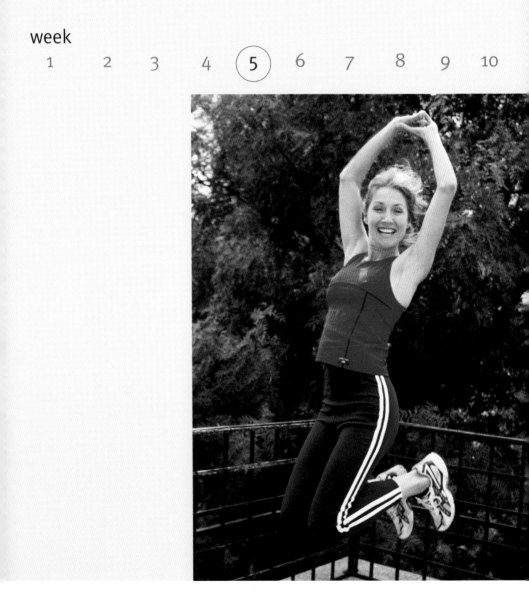

Week 5 planner

By this week, you are halfway through the programme, so don't give up! At this stage, you should be beginning to feel – and to see – some significant results.

Exercise

Your body is starting to take on a new look and you are feeling good about yourself. Do not give up on the relaxation treatments. You deserve them, so be good to yourself. Try to carry out your aerobic work in the morning or early afternoon; as you become fitter you could become overstimulated if you exercise aerobically last thing at night. This week sees the introduction of press-ups, which are wonderful for toning the upper arms and supporting the chest. Start with the easy press-ups and it will not be long before you can move on to the harder ones. Listen to your body when you exercise. If you feel it is too much, cut back on the number of repetitions.

Diet

If you are suffering any aches and pains, or the beginnings of a cold, make sure you eat some immune-boosting food. Raw vegetables, fruit, garlic and onions will all help. Make some leek and potato soup which is rich in vitamins A and C, potassium, iron, zinc, selenium and folic acid. Do not skip breakfast, even if you are starting to get out and about now. Your energy levels will plummet and you will be tempted to reach for a chocolate bar or another variety of high-sugar snack. Your body will work most effectively on a large breakfast, protein lunch and a light carbohydrate supper. While you are sleeping, the carbohydrates are broken down to release energy slowly.

WEEKLY PROGRESS CHART

Chart your progress on the 10-week recovery plan each week by making notes against these points. It will help you stay focused and motivated.

Date

Weight

How I feel about my appearance:

Skin

Hair

Weight loss

Muscle tone

Did I follow the diet plan this week?

Number of minutes/sets of exercises achieved this week

Monday

Warm-up	12 mins
Pelvic floor exercises	10 mins
Biceps curls	12 x 3 sets
Weighted triceps	12 x 3 sets
Roll-outs	12 x 3 sets
Buttock squeezes	12 x 3 sets
Hip flexor stretch	1 for each leg

RELAXATION: Salute to the Sun yoga pose after getting up or at the end of the day (see pages 76–77). Concentrate on using the breath.

TIP: Plan a day out with some girlfriends and babies, perhaps to a child-friendly restaurant or park. Write the date in your diary and go!

Tuesday

Warm-up	12 mins
Pelvic floor exercises	10 mins
Easy curl-ups	12 x 3 sets
Curl-downs	12 x 3 sets
Oblique curl-ups	12 x 3 sets
Cat stretch	

AEROBIC EXERCISE:15 minutes' marching; 2 minutes' step.
RELAXATION: Refining Body Scrub (see page 73).

TIP: If you have a rebounder, you can substitute this for or add it to your aerobic work. It is very beneficial for increasing stamina and taking weight off the legs.

Wednesday

Warm-up	12 mins
Pelvic floor exercises	12 mins
Waist-whittler	12 x 3 sets
Thigh kickbacks (see page 50)	12 x 3 sets
Buttock squeezes	12 x 3 sets
Hamstring stretch	3 for each leg

RELAXATION: Revitalizing Foot Spa (see page 82).

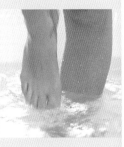

Thursday

Warm-up & Pelvic floor exercises	12 mins of each
Press-ups (see page 46)	8
Easy curl-ups	16 x 3 sets
Oblique curl-ups	16 x 3 sets
Curl-downs	16 x 3 sets
Inner thigh stretch	

AEROBIC EXERCISE: 7 minutes' marching; 6 minutes' step; 5 minutes' stair-climbing.
RELAXATION: T'ai chi – chi energy circulation movement. Stand with feet hip-width apart, knees bent. Relax your shoulders but keep your head lifted up, arms by your sides and away from your body. Shift your weight on to your right foot. Raise your arms up in front of you to shoulder height. Keep your palms and fingers pointing down. Immediately transfer your weight on to your left foot. In one flowing movement, lower your arms down to your sides and bend your wrists so that your hands are parallel to the floor. Move your weight back on to your right foot. Lift your arms in front of you to shoulder height. Repeat in one continuous sequence, moving easily.

TIP: List those telephone numbers that are important and pin them next to the phone along with a pen and paper, e.g. health visitor, doctor, and babysitter.

Friday

Warm-up	12 mins
Pelvic floor exercises	12 mins
Thigh kickbacks	16 x 3 sets
Doggies	12 x 3 sets
Inner thigh toner	16 x 3 sets
Leg lifts	16 x 3 sets
Weighted triceps	16 x 3 sets
Hamstring stretch	3 for each leg

RELAXATION: **Facial massage** (see page 79).

TIP: Burn some lavender essential oil in an essential oil burner in the baby's room before you put your baby down to sleep. Warning: Never leave a lit candle unattended.

Saturday

Warm-up	12 mins
Pelvic floor exercises	12 mins
Waist-whittler	12 x 3 sets
Cat stretch	
Easy curl-ups	16x 3 sets
Curl-downs	16 x 3 sets
Oblique curl-ups	16 x 3 sets
Hip flexor stretch	each leg

AEROBIC EXERCISE: 45 minutes' brisk walking.
RELAXATION: **Pedicure** plus **relaxing foot bath**. Place a couple of handfuls of pebbles in a bucket or washing-up bowl. Half-fill with warm water, then add a handful of sea salt, 1 drop marjoram essential oil blended with 1 teaspoon sweet almond oil, 1 drop pure peppermint essential oil and 1 drop lavender essential oil. Soak the feet while rolling the pebbles across the soles.

TIP: Make sure you are spending time with your partner alone. Have you planned a babysitter yet so that you can have a night out?

Sunday

Warm-up	12 mins
Pelvic floor exercises	12 mins
Press-ups	8 x 2 sets
Doggies	12 x 3 sets
Thigh kickbacks	16 x 3 sets
Cobra	
Biceps curls	16 x 3 sets
Inner thigh stretch	

RELAXATION: **Salute to the Sun yoga pose** (see page 76–77).

TIP: Stop worrying! What you need now is to laugh, so go and see a friend who makes you laugh or rent a video that does the same.

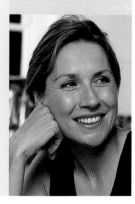

10-week plan

week

1   2   3   4   5   ⑥   7   8   9   10

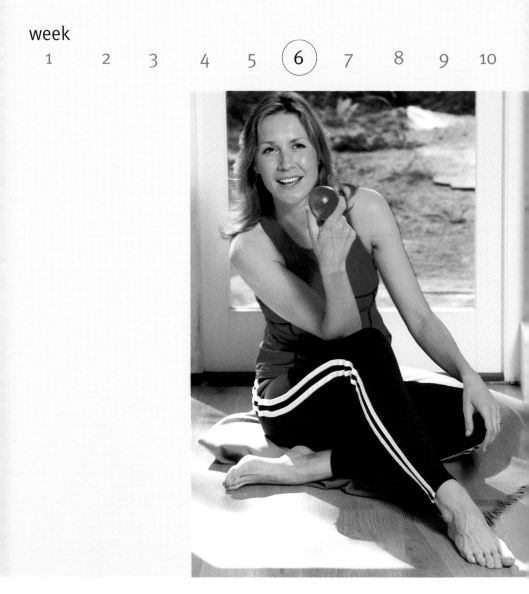

Week 6 planner

By this week of the programme you are starting to build strength and stamina all through your body, not just in your abdominals, which get a particular work-out this week.

Exercise

If your back or shoulders are aching when you are tired, watch how you are carrying and lifting your baby. All too often backs can be damaged through strain and stress from the birth and incorrect lifting techniques. When you get the opportunity, check your posture in front of the mirror. Remember to use the Checking Your Posture technique (see page 31) if you find that you are sitting slumped in your chair.

We will be working on the abdominals this week, making them stronger. A strong back is necessary for the stomach muscles to work well. If you find the crunchies too demanding, cut back and then build up again. Remember to exhale the breath each time you lift and contract up. Stomach muscles work when you concentrate on them.

Diet

Make sure that you are keeping up your intake of Vitamin B since this nourishes your overstretched nervous system. Include meat, poultry, fish, brown rice, milk and dried fruit in your diet. Also, if you are breast-feeding, keep up your calcium intake, since it is being used in your breastmilk.

Remind yourself that your diet should be healthy rather than calorie-controlled; you need all the nutrients for the body to perform effectively and to readjust to its new status. If you begin to feel deprived on the food front, find a recipe that you really enjoy as a treat and have a large portion of it at the end of the week. Add colour to your diet to keep it interesting and appealing, for example in the form of red peppers, green broccoli and yellow sweetcorn.

WEEKLY PROGRESS CHART

Chart your progress on the 10-week recovery plan each week by making notes against these points. It will help you stay focused and motivated.

Date _____

Weight _____

How I feel about my appearance:

Skin _____

Hair _____

Weight loss _____

Muscle tone _____

Did I follow the diet plan this week?

_____

_____

Number of minutes/sets of exercises achieved this week

_____

_____

week

Monday

Warm-up	10 mins
Pelvic floor exercises	15 mins
Crunchies (see page 42)	8
Oblique curl-ups	12 x 3 sets
Curl-downs	12 x 3 sets
Waist-whittler	12 x 3 sets
Inner thigh stretch	

AEROBIC EXERCISE: 20 minutes' marching or 10 minutes' dancing.
RELAXATION: **Meditation** (see page 74–75).

TIP: Share workout videos with a friend. Mix and match for effectiveness and economy.

Tuesday

Warm-up	10 mins
Pelvic floor exercises	15 mins
Biceps curls	12 x 3 sets
Weighted triceps	12 x 3 sets
Press-ups	8 x 3 sets
Roll-outs	12 x 3 sets
Hamstring stretch	3 for each leg

RELAXATION: **Breathing exercise** (see page 32).

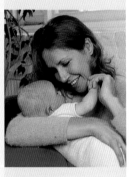

Wednesday

Warm-up	10 mins
Pelvic floor exercises	10 mins
Crunchies	12 x 3 sets
Easy curl-ups	12 x 3 sets
Oblique curl-ups	12 x 3 sets
Buttock squeezes	12 x 3 sets

AEROBIC EXERCISE: 2 minutes' jogging; 8 minutes' stair-climbing; 5 minutes' marching.
RELAXATION: **Hydrotherapy treatment** (see page 73).

TIP: If you are returning to work, check that your childcare arrangements are all in place.

Thursday

Warm-up	10 mins
Pelvic floor exercises	10 mins
Doggies	12 x 3 sets
Leg lifts	12 x 3 sets
Pliés	12 x 3 sets
Curl-downs	12 x 3 sets
Hip flexor stretch	1 for each leg

RELAXATION: **Purifying Face Mask** (see page 61).

TIP: Book an appointment with the hairdresser. If you are experiencing hair problems, give your hair a treatment (see page 66).

Friday

Warm-up	10 mins
Pelvic floor exercises	10 mins
Crunchies	8 x 3 sets
Cobra	
Cat stretch	
Press-ups	8 x 3 sets
Inner thigh stretch	

AEROBIC EXERCISE: 5 minutes' jogging; 10 minutes' marching.
RELAXATION: Dry skin brushing (see page 73); **hydrotherapy treatment** (see page 73).

TIP: Your body is starting to change shape again now, so why not buy a new outfit?

Saturday

Warm-up	10 mins
Pelvic floor exercises	10 mins
Leg lifts	12 x 3 sets
Pliés	12 x 3 sets
Waist-whittler	12 x 3 sets
Roll-outs	12 x 3 sets
Biceps curls	12 x 3 sets
Weighted triceps	12 x 3 sets
Hamstring stretch	3 for each leg

RELAXATION: Meditation (see pages 74–75).

TIP: If you are starting to wean your baby from the breast, you can cut excessive milk production by drinking a cup of sage tea night and morning.

Sunday

Warm-up	10 mins
Pelvic floor exercises	10 mins
Crunchies	12 x 3 sets
Curl-downs	12 x 3 sets
Small hip rolls	4
Hip flexor stretch	4
Cat stretch	

AEROBIC EXERCISE: 5 minutes' jogging; 10 minutes' stair-climbing or 10 minutes' step.
RELAXATION: Foot massage (see page 82).

TIP: For an instant lift at breakfast, try this drink. Blend 1 small banana and 2 ready-to-eat dried apricots, roughly chopped, ½ orange, peeled and pith removed, 1 kiwifruit, peeled, 1 teaspoon runny honey and 1 teaspoon wheatgerm in a food processor or blender. With the machine running, very slowly add 250 ml/8 fl oz skimmed cows' milk, soya or goats' milk until you have a frothy shake. Stir in 2 tablespoons natural bio yogurt and drink straight away.

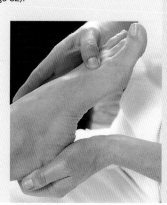

10-week plan

week

1   2   3   4   5   6   ⑦   8   9   10

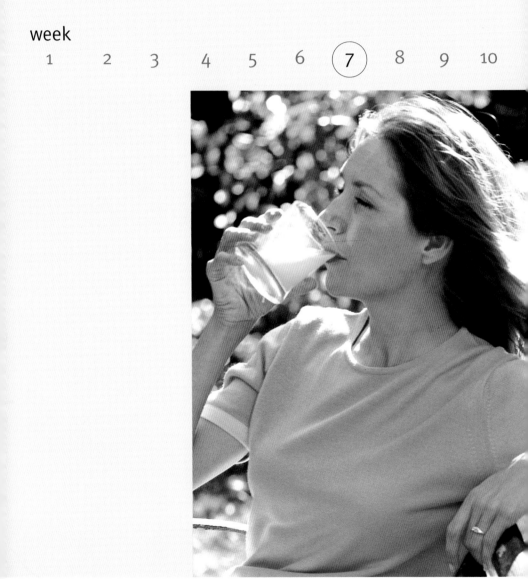

Week 7 planner

As you build up your aerobic work, consider joining an exercise class. It is sociable and will keep you motivated. Try to find one nearby that has a crèche or is run in the evening.

Exercise

Make sure that the instructor of your exercise class is well aware that you are returning to exercise after the birth of your baby. That way, if it is not a postnatal class, he or she can adapt some of the exercises for you. Do not be too ambitious; it is much better to start with a class that you feel is too easy and progress than find yourself in a high-impact aerobic class full of lean, toned bodies. A good pair of trainers is essential and will support not only your feet but your knees and hip joints, so go to a reputable sports shop.

Diet

Remember that fresh fruit and vegetable juices will provide you with instant energy boosts. Make one before your exercise session and drink it afterwards. Water, too, is important, particularly as you build up your aerobic capacity. Try to drink before, during and after exercise, and bear in mind that if you are thirsty, you are already dehydrated. Eat some cherry tomatoes to revitalize your skin; they are packed with vitamins and antioxidants. You can also feed your skin externally by applying a face mask (see page 68).

WEEKLY PROGRESS CHART

Chart your progress on the 10-week recovery plan each week by making notes against these points. It will help you stay focused and motivated.

Date _____

Weight _____

How I feel about my appearance:

Skin _____

Hair _____

Weight loss _____

Muscle tone _____

Did I follow the diet plan this week?

_____

_____

Number of minutes/sets of exercises achieved this week

_____

_____

1   2   3   4   5   6   (7)   8   9   10

Monday

Warm-up	10 mins
Pelvic floor exercises	10 mins
Lunges (see page 51)	8
Leg lifts	12 x 3 sets
Easy curl-ups	12 x 3 sets
Buttock squeezes	12 x 3 sets

RELAXATION: **Revitalizing Foot Spa** (see page 82).

TIP: If your baby has been immunized, try the local swimming pool. There may even be a class for new babies and the chance to meet some different people.

Tuesday

Warm-up	10 mins
Pelvic floor exercises	10 mins
Waist-whittler	12 x 3 sets
Small hip rolls	6
Hip flexor stretch	
Thigh kickbacks	12 x 3 sets
Hamstring stretch	3 for each leg

AEROBIC EXERCISE: 15 minutes' marching or 10 minutes' dancing.
RELAXATION: **Stimulating scalp oil and massage** (see page 66).

TIP: If you are planning a weekend away with your partner and baby, make a list of items to take and find out what might be supplied.

Wednesday

Warm-up	10 mins
Pelvic floor exercises	10 mins
Crunchies	12 x 3 sets
Curl-downs	12 x 3 sets
Cat stretch	
Roll-outs	12 x 3 sets
Biceps curls	12 x 3 sets
Doggies	12 x 3 sets
Hip flexor stretch	1 for each leg

RELAXATION: **Aromatherapy bath** – add a few drops of lavender, geranium and mandarin essential oils to the water for a soothing bath.

TIP: Date and file all those photographs you took of your new arrival. Babies change so quickly that you will soon forget how old they really were at the time – and how small!

Thursday

Warm-up	10 mins
Pelvic floor exercises	10 mins
Lunges	8 x 2 sets
Press-ups	12 x 3 sets
Roll-outs	12 x 3 sets
Waist-whittlers	12 x 3 sets
Cobra	
Inner thigh stretch	

AEROBIC EXERCISE: 10 minutes' stair-climbing; 5 minutes' jogging.
RELAXATION: **T'ai chi** – chi energy circulation movement (see page 104).

TIP: You could increase your aerobic exercise by walking more. If you are taking the baby, invest in a rucksack as a handbag. They are not only fashionable but practical.

Friday

Warm-up	10 mins
Pelvic floor exercises	10 mins
Crunchies	12 x 3 sets
Easy curl-ups	12 x 3 sets
Oblique curl-ups	16 x 3 sets
Triceps dips (see page 48)	8
Cat stretch	
Hip flexor stretch	

RELAXATION: Facial massage (see page 79).

TIP: Try dancing again. Put on some music and let rip in the lounge – a particularly good idea if it is a cold, rainy day. It will make you feel better, too.

Saturday

Warm-up	10 mins
Pelvic floor exercises	10 mins
Cat stretch	
Waist-whittler	12 x 3 sets
Thigh kickbacks	12 x 3 sets
Inner thigh stretch	

AEROBIC EXERCISE: 10 minutes' jogging; 5 minutes' skipping.
RELAXATION: Foot massage (see page 82).

TIP: Go along to a beauty counter at your local pharmacy and get them to give you a makeover. Some companies need you to book, but others are happy to do it immediately.

Sunday

Warm-up	10 mins
Pelvic floor exercises	10 mins
Press-ups	12 x 3 sets
Triceps dips	8 x 2 sets
Leg lifts	12 x 3 sets
Pliés	12 x 3 sets
Buttock squeezes	12 x 3 sets
Hamstring stretch	3 for each leg

RELAXATION: Back massage (see page 79).

TIP: Try this delicious mango and peach revitalizer. Peel, stone and roughly chop 1 peach and 1 mango. Blend in a food processor or blender until smooth. Add 5 tablespoons orange juice, 150 ml/¼ pint low-fat yogurt and 2 teaspoons pouring honey and blend. This is a wonderful combination for healthy skin, hair, nails and eyes since it is rich in the antioxidant vitamins A and C as well as metabolism-boosting iodine and calcium.

10-week plan

week

1   2   3   4   5   6   7   (8)   9   10

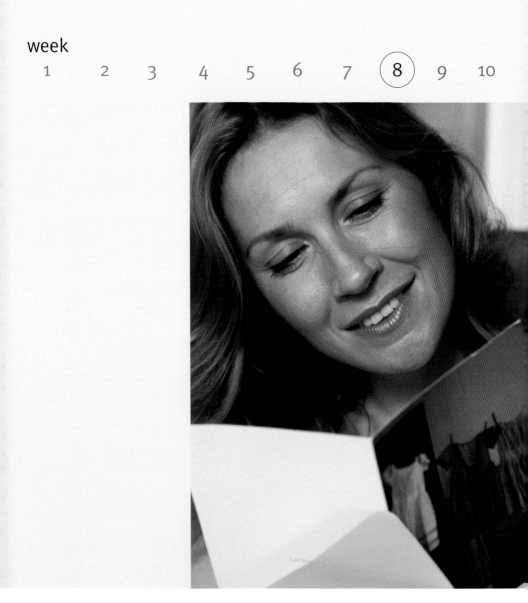

Week 8 planner

If you can, try cycling – it will improve your cardiovascular system and tone your thighs. When the baby is old enough, you can have a baby seat put on to the back of your cycle.

Exercise

Swimming is another useful aerobic exercise and the water will ease any aches you may have, so see if you can attend your local pool on a regular basis. Practise your yoga poses (see pages 76–77 and 93) since these will stretch your body and bring relief to aches and pains. Is your baby getting heavy in the sling – is it time to buy the next size sling?

Remember to breathe fully into your abdomen when you are working on any of the relaxation methods. If you find that you are getting stressed when shopping or behind the wheel of the car, use these techniques then as well.

Diet

You are probably finding that you are starting to cut back on the number of meals. If not, do not worry – your body is your best adviser. If you need food to restore energy levels, then try to keep the plate sizes small and watch that you do not add any unnecessary fat, such as salad dressings or an extra-thick spreading of butter on bread. If you have cut back and find that you suddenly become hungry, go back to keeping some easy-to-nibble healthy snacks in the refrigerator and in the storecupboard. A glass of wine may be enjoyable in the evening at the weekend or when you are both relaxing, but if you are breast-feeding, ensure that you keep alcohol levels to a minimum.

WEEKLY PROGRESS CHART

Chart your progress on the 10-week recovery plan each week by making notes against these points. It will help you stay focused and motivated.

Date _____

Weight _____

How I feel about my appearance:

Skin _____

Hair _____

Weight loss _____

Muscle tone _____

Did I follow the diet plan this week?

_____

_____

Number of minutes/sets of exercises achieved this week

_____

_____

Monday

Warm-up	10 mins
Breathing and posture	5 mins
Pelvic floor exercises	15 mins
Crunchies	12 x 3 sets
Extended obliques (see page 43)	8
Cobra	
Thigh kickbacks	12 x 3 sets
Inner thigh stretch	

AEROBIC EXERCISE: 20 minutes' marching.
RELAXATION: **Aromatherapy bath** (see page 72).

TIP: Try to increase the amount of aerobic exercise you are taking to 20 minutes three times per week.

Tuesday

Warm-up	10 mins
Pelvic floor exercises	15 mins
Biceps curls with weights (see page 47)	8 x 3 sets
Overhead triceps curls (see page 47)	8 x 3 sets
Small hip rolls	4
Buttock squeezes	12 x 3 sets
Hip flexor stretch	1 for each leg

RELAXATION: **Home Spa Bath** (see page 72).

TIP: If you suffer from cystitis or any other urinary infections, try drinking cranberry juice. It helps stop the bacteria clinging to the urinary tract.

Wednesday

Warm-up	10 mins
Pelvic floor exercises	15 mins
Waist-whittler	12 x 3 sets
Inner thigh toner	12 x 3 sets
Leg lifts	12 x 3 sets
Hamstring stretch	3 for each leg

AEROBIC EXERCISE: 15 minutes' jogging.
RELAXATION: **Refining Body Scrub** (see page 73).

TIP: For chapped hands, mix a few drops of glycerine with a couple of drops of lemon essential oil. Massage into your hands at bedtime.

Thursday

Warm-up	10 mins
Pelvic floor exercises	15 mins
Cobra	
Press-ups	12 x 3 sets
Triceps dips	12 x 3 sets
Crunchies	12 x 3 sets

RELAXATION: **Meditation** (see pages 74–75).

TIP: Check your contraception. If you are breast-feeding, you may not be having periods, but this does not necessarily mean you cannot become pregnant.

Friday

Warm-up	10 mins
Pelvic floor exercises	15 mins
Overhead triceps curls	8 x 2 sets
Biceps curls with weights	8 x 2 sets
Roll-outs	8 x 2 sets
Doggies	12 x 3 sets
Crunchies	12 x 3 sets
Hamstring stretch	3 for each leg

AEROBIC EXERCISE: 10 minutes' jogging; 5 minutes' skipping; 5 minutes' stair-climbing.
RELAXATION: Reflexology (see page 83).

TIP: It is time to buy a skipping rope. Choose one from a sports shop since this will be strong enough to last.

Saturday

Warm-up	10 mins
Pelvic floor exercises	15 mins
Crunchies	12 x 3 sets
Curl-downs	12 x 3 sets
Extended obliques	12 x 3 sets
Pliés	12 x 3 sets
Buttock squeezes	12 x 3 sets
Inner thigh stretch	

RELAXATION: Anti-cellulite massage (see page 81).

TIP: Try a cup of raspberry leaf tea. While helpful during the end of pregnancy, it is also good for healing, restoring and balancing the uterus. You can make your own infusion or buy raspberry leaf tea bags from a health shop.

Sunday

Warm-up	10 mins
Pelvic floor exercises	15 mins
Cat stretch	
Lunges	12 x 3 sets
Inner thigh toner	12 x 3 sets
Hip flexor stretch	4
Leg lifts	12 x 3 sets
Triceps dips	12 x 3 sets

AEROBIC EXERCISE: 1 hour's walking or 10 minutes' step; 5 minutes' jogging.
RELAXATION: Salute to the Sun yoga pose (see page 76–77).

TIP: Eat some liquorice. It helps support the adrenal glands, fights infection and is good if you find yourself suffering from lack of sleep.

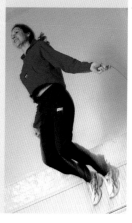

10-week plan

week

1   2   3   4   5   6   7   8   ⑨   10

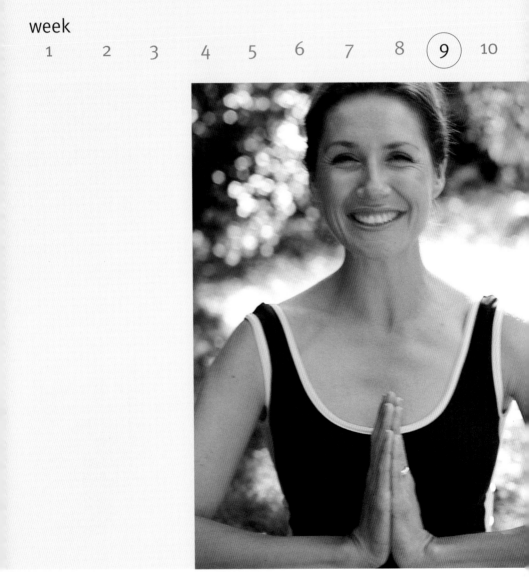

Week 9 planner

You have suddenly discovered that your aerobic work has increased, but you can go on longer without becoming short of breath.

Exercise

You are stronger than before and more toned now. With this new you staring you in the face, you want to show it off, so find somewhere to go and enjoy yourselves for the evening. Social exercise, such as dancing, is great fun and also helps build fitness. If your pelvic floor is being put to the test, then try to increase the amount of times you work on it during the day. Take your time with the pelvic floor exercises. You need control over all the muscles to make them work efficiently. Pulling them up and letting them go straight away will not tighten them significantly. It is the slow, controlled movements that pull them together. You will always need these muscles, so make sure you work them now.

Diet

The end of the plan is in sight and you cannot only see a difference but also feel it. If you need warming food to start off the day, try porridge oats. They are low in fat but also highly nutritious. Now that you have begun to eat healthily, you may find that your tastebuds have changed. Try to think of this as a new way of eating for life, a healthy lifestyle and a healthy you. Once you begin to introduce solids to your baby's diet, you can look to your own plate for inspiration and ideas first. Organic produce is best and will give your child a good start in life. You may also find that your baby has fewer allergies or adverse reactions to these foods since they are free of preservatives and pesticides.

WEEKLY PROGRESS CHART

Chart your progress on the 10-week recovery plan each week by making notes against these points. It will help you stay focused and motivated.

Date

Weight

How I feel about my appearance:

Skin

Hair

Weight loss

Muscle tone

Did I follow the diet plan this week?

Number of minutes/sets of exercises achieved this week

Monday

Warm-up	10 mins
Breathing and posture	5 minutes
Pelvic floor exercises	15 mins
Cat stretch	
Cobra	
Press-ups	8 x 3 sets
Extended obliques	12 x 3 sets
Crunchies	16 x 3 sets

AEROBIC EXERCISE: 5 minutes' skipping twice per day or for 10 minutes once per day.
RELAXATION: **Breathing exercise** (see page 32).

TIP: Keep your plate size small but topped up, particularly if you are still eating several meals a day.

Tuesday

Warm-up	10 mins
Pelvic floor exercises	15 mins
Pliés	12 x 3 sets
Leg lifts	16 x 3 sets
Buttock squeezes	16 x 3 sets

RELAXATION: **Refreshing Bath Gel** (see page 73).

TIP: Do not drink tea or coffee with your lunch since they contain caffeine and tannins that interfere with iron absorption.

Wednesday

Warm-up	10 minutes
Pelvic floor exercises	15 minutes
Cobra	
Cat stretch	
Hamstring stretch	4 for each leg

AEROBIC EXERCISE: 7 minutes' skipping; 5 minutes' stair-climbing.
RELAXATION: **Back massage** – try the Sensual Massage Oil (see page 78); **Salute to the Sun yoga pose** (see page 76–77).

TIP: For a treat, try meringue topped with raspberries and organic yogurt for dessert. Although sumptuously sweet, it is low in fat and healthy – the ideal comfort food.

Thursday

Warm-up	10 mins
Breathing and posture	5 mins
Pelvic floor exercises	15 mins
Overhead triceps curls	12 x 3 sets
Biceps curls with weights	12 x 3 sets
Press-ups	12 x 3 sets
Hip flexor stretch	each leg

RELAXATION: **Scalp massage** (see page 66).

TIP: Check your posture in the mirror (see page 31) and try to be conscious about the way you sit. Breathe into your lower chest and abdomen three times today for five minutes and see how you feel.

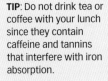

Friday

Warm-up	10 mins
Pelvic floor exercises	15 mins
Crunchies	16 x 3 sets
Buttock squeezes	12 x 3 sets
Extended obliques	12 x 3 sets
Thigh kickbacks	12 x 3 sets
Inner thigh stretch	

AEROBIC EXERCISE: 7 minutes' skipping; 5 minutes' marching.
RELAXATION: Meditation (see page 74–75).

TIP: Invest in a water filter for the home. There are many available on the market and it will work out cheaper than bottled water. You do not have to keep it in the refrigerator; water drunk at room temperature is better for you than cold water.

Saturday

Warm-up	10 mins
Pelvic floor exercises	15 mins
Lunges	12 x 3 sets
Overhead triceps curls	12 x 3 sets
Biceps curls with weights	12 x 3 sets
Extended obliques	12 x 3 sets
Cobra	
Hamstring stretch	4 for each leg

RELAXATION: Float Like a Cloud T'ai chi sequence of slow, graceful, continuous movements – stand with feet shoulder-width apart, knees slightly bent and arms by your sides. Gently shift your weight on to your right foot and raise the left arm to shoulder height. Keep the fingers of the left arm pointing down. Keep your right arm by your side and bend the wrist so that it is parallel to the floor. Shift your weight to your left foot and raise your right arm to shoulder height, fingers pointing down. Keep the left arm by your side and bend the wrist so that your hand is parallel to the floor. Repeat each side twice more. This exercise aids circulation, exercises muscles, deepens breathing and stimulates the blood and lymph circulation.

TIP: Nutmeg warms the digestive system. Grate a little from a whole nutmeg over winter greens, spinach, cabbage or broccoli.

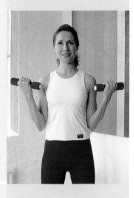

Sunday

Warm-up	10 mins
Pelvic floor exercises	15 mins
Breathing and posture	5 mins
Press-ups	12 x 3 sets
Thigh kickbacks	12 x 3 sets
Leg lifts	12 x 3 sets
Triceps dips	12 x 3 sets
Hip flexor stretch	1 for each leg

AEROBIC EXERCISE: 5 minutes' stair-climbing; 5 minutes' skipping; 10 minutes' step.
RELAXATION: Aromatherapy bath (see page 72).

TIP: Share your baby – both sets of grandparents will love to help and to see you.

10-week plan

1   2   3   4   5   6   7   8   9   (10)

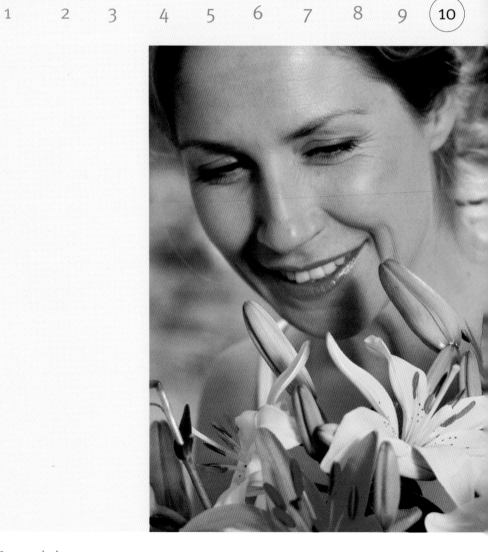

Week 10 planner

You have now reached the final week of the 10-week recovery plan which I am sure seemed a lifetime away when you started nine weeks ago.

Exercise

If there are any exercises that you have not managed to keep up with, this is the week to work away at them. If you want to, you can increase the number of repetitions to make them harder. You can now add the exercises with your baby if you need a heavier weight or if your baby is more awake and does not want you to exercise (see pages 56–59). It is not a case, though, of thinking once this week is finished, that is it. Unfortunately, fitness cannot be stored so you will need to keep on.

By now you will have some idea of what you like doing and how motivated you are. Find a friend to keep you company in your exercising if you need the extra push and remember that fitness is important in your life because it keeps you healthy. As a mother, you will realize that you do not have the time to be ill any more. Exercise will help ward off those illnesses and viruses, maintaining your body for the next baby to come!

Diet

Hopefully you will be shopping healthily by now. Use a shopping list if it helps and stick to it. Do not be tempted to buy those chocolate biscuits because they are cheaper this week. Put the money towards a beauty treatment instead. Try not to shop when you are hungry – this really is a recipe for disaster and all your good intentions will go out of the window. Experiment with herbs and natural flavours. How about growing some herbs on the windowsill or planting a herb garden? You can use them in your face packs and baths as well as in cooking. Make sure that you eat oily fish, such as salmon, mackerel and sardines, twice a week if possible, since it is high in unsaturated oils and omega-3 fatty acids, which are highly beneficial to health.

If you are experiencing any stomach bloating or fluid retention, look to your diet first. Keep a record to see when the bloating occurs and try natural diuretics, such as celery, for fluid retention. Then look in the mirror. Does your hair not gleam and your skin seem fresh? You not only feel well but look good, too!

WEEKLY PROGRESS CHART

Chart your progress on the 10-week recovery plan each week by making notes against these points. It will help you stay focused and motivated.

Date _____

Weight _____

How I feel about my appearance:

Skin _____

Hair _____

Weight loss _____

Muscle tone _____

Did I follow the diet plan this week?

_____

_____

Number of minutes/sets of exercises achieved this week

_____

_____

week

Monday

Warm-up	10 mins
Pelvic floor exercises	15 mins
Inner thigh toner	12 x 3 sets
Leg lifts	12 x 3 sets
Crunchies	16 x 3 sets
Hamstring stretch	4 for each leg

RELAXATION: **Refining Body Scrub and Body Lotion** (see page 73).

TIP: Take your shoes off and give your feet an airing. Walk around the house barefoot as much as you can.

Tuesday

Warm-up	10 mins
Pelvic floor exercises	15 mins
Crunchies	12 x 3 sets
Extended obliques	12 x 3 sets
Inner thigh stretch	12 x 3 sets
Thigh kickbacks	12 x 3 sets
Hip flexor stretch	1 for each leg

AEROBIC EXERCISE: 10 minutes' skipping; 10 minutes' step.
RELAXATION: **Reflexology** (see page 83).

TIP: Try this mini liver cleanser. Mix together 1 tablespoon olive oil, 1 crushed garlic clove, 1 cm/½ piece of grated fresh root ginger, juice of 1 lemon and apple juice to taste. Enjoy!

Wednesday

Warm-up	10 mins
Breathing and posture	5 mins
Pelvic floor exercises	15 mins
Lunges	12 x 3 sets
Press-ups	12 x 3 sets
Biceps curls with weights	12 x 3 sets
Overhead triceps curls	12 x 3 sets
Roll-outs	12 x 3 sets
Small hip rolls	4
Inner thigh stretch	

RELAXATION: **Meditation** (see page 74–75).

TIP: Take advantage of the packing help at supermarkets. If no one offers, ask for some help and with carrying your shopping to the car. Now that the baby is growing, you must look after your back.

Thursday

Warm-up	10 mins
Pelvic floor exercises	15 mins
Cat stretch	
Cobra	
Leg lifts	16 x 3 sets
Inner thigh toner	12 x 3 sets
Leg lifts	12 x 3 sets
Thigh kickbacks	16 x 3 sets
Crunchies	16 x 3 sets
Triceps dips	12 x 3 sets
Inner thigh stretch	

AEROBIC EXERCISE: 10 minutes' stair-climbing; 5 minutes' step; 5 minutes' skipping.
RELAXATION: Have an **anti-cellulite massage** for kick-starting those tough areas (see page 81).

TIP: Check your health insurance for yourself, your partner and your baby. Also, check the arrangements concerning your mortgage and other insurances. It is time to consider making a will if you have not already done so.

week

1 2 3 4 5 6 7 8 9 (10)

Friday

Warm-up	10 mins
Pelvic floor exercises	15 mins
Lunges	12 x 3 sets
Leg lifts	16 x 3 sets
Crunchies	16 x 3 sets
Extended obliques	16 x 3 sets
Inner thigh toner	12 x 3 sets
Hamstring stretch	4 for each leg

RELAXATION: **Hydrotherapy treatment** (see page 73).

TIP: Fresh air is good for you and the baby. If you are using a push chair, make sure the handles are high enough, or get them adjusted so that they are.

Saturday

Warm-up	10 mins
Pelvic floor exercises	15 mins
Waist-whittler	12 x 3 sets
Press-ups	12 x 3 sets
Lunges	12 x 3 sets
Leg lifts	12 x 3 sets
Crunchies	16 x 3 sets
Hip flexor stretch	1 for each leg

AEROBIC EXERCISE: 1 hour's brisk walk or 15 minutes' jogging; 5 minutes' skipping.
RELAXATION: **Facial massage** (see page 79).

TIP: Try not to shop when you are hungry – this is a recipe for disaster!

Sunday

Warm-up	10 mins
Pelvic floor exercises	15 mins
Crunchies	16 x 3 sets
Press-ups	12 x 3 sets
Lunges	12 x 3 sets
Biceps curls with weights	12 x 3 sets
Triceps dips	12 x 3 sets
Hamstring stretch	4 for each leg

AEROBIC EXERCISE: 10 minutes' skipping; 10 minutes' jogging or rebounder.

RELAXATION: **Back massage** (see page 79).

TIP: You can start exercising with your baby now if you find that she is awake a lot more. Be careful how you balance her and do not do anything that makes you feel uncomfortable. But you are now on your way – congratulations! Treat yourself to a new piece of workout wear or outfit. Keep it up!

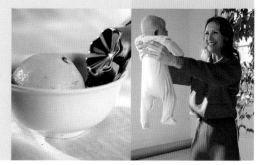

Index

Acknowledgements

**Octopus Publishing Group
Limited**/ Gary Latham 23, 24, 71
bottom centre, 96, 125 bottom
centre, /Peter Myers 13, 16 top, 21,
78, /Emma Peios 16 centre right,
/Peter Pugh-Cook 1, 3, 6, 7, 8, 9,
10, 11, 14, 15, 17 centre right, 20,
26, 27, 28, 29, 31, 33, 34, 35, 36 top
left, 36 centre, 36 top right, 36
bottom, 37 top, 37 centre, 37
bottom, 38 top left, 38 top right, 38
bottom, 39 top left, 39 top right, 39
bottom right, 39 bottom left, 40, 40
top left, 40 bottom, 41, 41 top left,
41 top right, 41 bottom right, 42
top, 42 centre, 42 bottom, 43 top,
43 centre, 43 bottom, 44 top, 44
centre, 44 bottom, 45 top, 45
bottom right, 45 bottom left, 46
centre left, 46 top right, 46 centre
right, 46 bottom left, 47 top centre,
47 top left, 47 bottom right, 47
bottom centre, 48 top left, 48 top
right, 48 bottom right, 48 bottom
centre, 49 top, 49 bottom, 50 top,
50 bottom, 51 left, 51 right, 52 left,
52 right, 53 top, 53 centre, 53
bottom, 54 top, 54 centre, 54
bottom, 55 top, 55 centre, 55
bottom, 56 top, 56 bottom, 57 top,
57 bottom, 58 left, 58 right, 59 top,
59 bottom, 60, 61, 62, 63, 64, 65,
66, 67, 68, 72, 75, 76, 77, 79, 80, 81,
82 left, 82 right, 83, 84, 86, 89
bottom centre, 90, 94, 98, 101, 102,
105, 106, 108, 109, 110, 113, 114,
117, 118, 120, 121, 122, 125,
/William Reavell 12, 17 top right, 71
bottom right, 71 bottom left, 89
bottom right, 93, /Ian Wallace 73,
85, 104, /Mark Winwood 18, 19.

Executive Editor – Jane McIntosh
Editor – Sharon Ashman
Senior Designer – Rozelle Bentheim
Book Design – Lisa Tai
Picture Researcher – Jennifer Veall
Senior Production Controller– Jo Sim